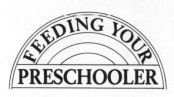

Also by Louise Lambert-Lagacé

Feeding Your Baby in the Nineties

The Nutrition Challenge for Women

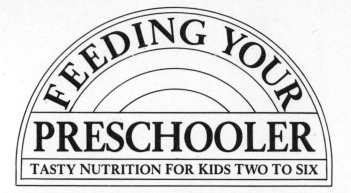

FEEDING YOUR PRESCHOOLER

TASTY NUTRITION FOR KIDS TWO TO SIX

LOUISE LAMBERT-LAGACÉ

Stoddart

First published in 1993 by
Stoddart Publishing Co. Limited
34 Lesmill Road
Toronto, Canada
M3B 2T6
(416) 445-3333

Canadian Cataloguing in Publication Data

Lambert-Lagacé, Louise, 1941-
Feeding your pre-schooler

Includes bibliographical references and index.
ISBN 0-7737-5588-8

1. Children – Nutrition. 1. Infants – nutrition.
I. Title.

RJ206.L35 1993   649'.3   C93-094054-7

Cover design: Gillian Stead
Cover photograph: Peter Paterson
Text design: Brant Cowie/ArtPlus Limited
Printed and bound in Canada

Some of the material in this book originally appeared in La Sage bouffe de 2 à 6 ans by the same author, published by Les Éditions de l'Homme in 1984.

Note: The information contained in this book is presented as a guide. For specific medical problems consult your physician.

Stoddart Publishing gratefully acknowledges the support of the Canada Council, the Ontario Ministry of Culture, Tourism, and Recreation, Ontario Arts Council, and Ontario Publishing Centre in the development of writing and publishing in Canada.

Contents

Acknowledgements

FEEDING YOUR PRESCHOOLER was not written in isolation. A number of exceptional dietitians helped me put this book together:

Sheila Dubois systematically reviewed the scientific literature dealing with all aspects of the preschooler's development for the original French edition. Her insight and extensive efforts made my work so much easier.

Lison Chauvin-Desourdy, mother of three preschoolers, helped me develop recipes and gave me excellent comments all through the project.

Cynthia Dougherty and Suzette Poliquin collected information, calculated menus, and reviewed the manuscript.

Mary Bush surveyed a group of parents at Algonquin College, Deanne Delaney surveyed parents at the outpatient clinic of the Montreal Children's Hospital, while Micheline Colin did the same at Saint Justine's Hospital.

More recently, Josée Thibodeau, my research assistant, and Caroline Marcoux, dietetic intern, reviewed the most recent articles of the scientific literature. We wanted to give answers to real problems and to provide practical yet proven methods of intervention.

Then Elsha Leventis at Stoddart did a superb job of editing and beautified the manuscript.

I thank them all most sincerely. I also wish to thank my husband, who, once more, let me work weekends and nights to complete this project.

Introduction

YOUR DREAM IS to have a healthy child who is hungry at every meal, who gobbles down every food you offer, and who always eats every morsel on his or her plate. Why should you have to sell food with songs and promises?

In reality, however, toddlers and preschoolers may have the appetite of a bird one day and eat like a horse the next. Quite a challenge for parents and caregivers!

The way you tackle your child's eating behavior can lead to the dream, or to a nightmare. A rigid approach can negatively affect your child's relationship with food, while a more flexible one can save a lot of aggravation and worry.

I wrote this book to provide a continuum to *Feeding Your Baby in the Nineties* (Stoddart, 1992). Feeding problems are quite different at 30 months than they were at six months, but your philosophy must be to continue to respect your child's needs at all times. The issues of quality and quantity remain important. If your baby was exposed to the most healthful foods during the first 18 months, this is no time to give up or to give in to second class foods. Although those first foods were critical for the baby's development, they do not provide lifelong protection against poor eating habits. Healthful eating must continue despite the many eating challenges preschool years provide.

I want to give you more than strategies to empty plates. My goal is to help you generate happy and healthy eaters. So many adults have eating problems that originate in childhood: perhaps they were repeatedly forced to eat, or nobody enjoyed eating around them, or calorie-rich foods were the main items on the menu. I am convinced that the prevention of most eating problems begins in the high chair simply by respecting the individuality of your child and by enjoying wholesome foods together.

In part one we'll look at your child's needs and whims to give you a better understanding of what goes on in the mind, heart, and body of your youngster when it comes to food. Do not worry if your child does not behave exactly according to this book. All children have their own eating styles and develop at their own pace.

In part two I look at a number of health problems that have food remedies. You'll find basic information on such conditions as constipation, obesity, and lactose intolerance and learn some simple, edible solutions. When dealing with a health problem, follow the suggested strategy with the collaboration of your family physician, or other health practitioner, who knows your child and his environment.

The information in part three answers all your questions about cooking techniques and hot issues such as hidden sugars, salt, or fats, issues that affect your meal plans and your child's food choices.

Part four contains lots of delicious recipes, from breakfast ideas to desserts, that take into account common food allergies and provide you with nutritional values.

In the appendixes you'll find charts of all the best sources of vitamins and minerals, as well as available supplements.

May this book help you develop the positive eating strategies that will turn your child into a lifelong happy eater.

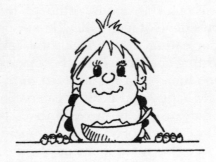

PART 1

The Needs and Whims of Young Children

Happy hearts and happy faces
Happy play in grassy places
That was how, in ancient ages,
Children grew to kings and sages.

ROBERT LOUIS STEVENSON,
   A Child's Garden of Verses

Too few of us, perhaps, feel that the breaking of bread, the sharing of salt,
the common dipping into one bowl, mean more than satisfaction of a need.

M. F. K. FISHER,
   The Art of Eating

Chapter One

The Preschooler's Eating Habits

THE EATING HABITS of toddlers and preschoolers are fascinating because children progress so rapidly from breast milk or formula to full, balanced diets. Along the way, the always-hungry baby may become a good eater or a fussy one. In fact, surveys show that *one child in four* systematically refuses food.

Naturally, parents worry that their children are not eating enough, but concerns about quantity can distract from the nutritional *quality* of a child's diet. The latest survey done in the United States among children aged two to ten compared their eating habits in 1988 with those in 1978 and concluded that their average intake of calories, fats, and carbohydrates remained constant while their daily vitamin and mineral intake was lower. In addition,

- 80 percent of children had inadequate intakes of zinc;
- More than 50 percent lacked calcium and vitamin B_6;
- 25 percent of children lacked iron and vitamin A.

Lately, the controversy surrounding fat, cholesterol, and sodium has led to a shift in food choices; it has reduced milk consumption, for instance, and has had a negative impact on the overall nutritional quality of foods children eat. But wholesome foods are available, and children's diets can be improved.

Today's children will likely spend at least some time in a day-care center, but parents and caregivers can still ensure that meals and snacks add up to a high quality diet.

Eventually, children do enjoy a variety of foods that reflect family and cultural preferences, but individual likes and dislikes exist even among preschoolers. A study carried out in a thousand American homes a few years ago revealed the following information:

- Children do not necessarily enjoy the same foods adults do and food preferences change over the years;
- Corn, carrots, and pickles were at the top of the list of favorite vegetables;
- Favorite fruits were grapes, apples, strawberries, and melon;

• Favorite desserts were ice cream, doughnuts, and chocolate chip cookies.

The last Canada-wide nutrition survey, dating back to the early 1970s, still provides relevant information on eating trends among preschoolers, such as the following classics:

• Preschoolers eat more cooked cereals than dry ones;
• They willingly accept whole wheat bread;
• They prefer ground meat over other cuts of meat;
• They enjoy sauces, chicken noodle soup, and desserts made with gelatine.

Meanwhile Mexican preschoolers enjoy chili peppers!

Culture influences a child's favorite-food list, but parents and care-takers have a crucial role to play in shaping the list, in linking *tasty* foods with nutritious foods. Research has shown that the more positive you are about cooking and eating wholesome foods, the healthier your child's diet will be.

You really can help shape the food culture of tomorrow!

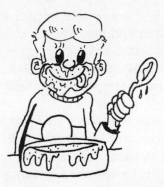

Chapter Two

Your Child's Nutritional Needs

BABIES GROW RAPIDLY, at an average rate of 9 percent per month, but when they reach their second birthday, the rate drops to about 1 percent growth per month. The type of weight gain is also different; a baby lays down body *fat*, requiring tons of calories, while the preschooler accumulates a higher proportion of *lean tissue*, which requires less calories. Preschoolers *need only half as many calories to gain a gram of weight* as do children under the age of two.

An important study published in the *New England Journal of Medicine* shows that erratic eating patterns can be considered normal for a preschooler. A child does not always eat the same amount of food, and a large meal often compensates for a lighter one. The total daily intake remains relatively constant for one child, but some preschoolers take in 1800 calories each day while others develop normally with 1100! Comparing big eaters and light eaters can cause a lot of needless distress, so relax!

The greatest challenge in feeding a preschooler is learning to respect the individual child rather than imposing recommended intakes in order to meet nutritional needs. Children of the same age, weight, and height, with similar levels of physical activity, do not necessarily have the same nutritional needs. So when I refer to a list of recommended nutrients, for example the Recommended Nutrient Intakes (RNIs) established by the Canadian government, these figures are only points of reference — tools to evaluate the quality of a diet for a group of preschoolers or to detect a possible deficiency. I have presented these recommendations (see Appendix A, pages 187–203) only to complement the information given and to reassure you, not to create new doubts or worries.

If you consult an American book, you may be surprised by the differences between Canadian recommended amounts and those published in the United States; but keep in mind that each set of recommendations only reflects the philosophy of a particular group of experts. Unanimity among experts is not common.

Take vitamin C, for instance. If you study the Canadian RNIs on page 000, you will see that the RNI for vitamin C is 20 milligrams per day at age two or three. We know that 20 milligrams of vitamin C exceeds the amount needed to prevent scurvy, the deficiency disease caused by a lack of vitamin C. We also know that in principle 20 milligrams meets the needs of 97.5 percent of healthy two- and three-year-olds. We also know that 30 milligrams may be insufficient for two or three children out of 100 or for a sick child.

If a healthy child consumes only 16 milligrams of vitamin C per day instead of 20 milligrams, he is not deficient, but the risk of becoming deficient increases if the daily intake falls below 50 percent of the recommended intake. There may be true vitamin C deficiency if the child has such symptoms as fatigue, weakness, small hemorrhages at the hair roots, muscular pain, swelling of the joints, and bleeding gums, but this kind of problem is extremely rare in Canada.

Offer your child the most nutritious foods every day, and stop worrying about the exact quantities of vitamins, proteins, or minerals. An occasional lapse won't affect the nutritional status of your child *if he eats well on a regular basis*.

It is your child's *growth and weight* curves that tell the real story, not the amount of calories or vitamins he swallows. If your child develops well and maintains a regular growth curve, he is probably getting enough of everything. Conversely, if there is a deviation in the normal curve in one direction or the other, he may be getting too many or too few nutrients for his needs.

To meet the nutritional needs of your preschooler, offer the most nutritious foods and let her determine the quantity. With this approach, your child stands a good chance of obtaining even more vitamins, proteins, and minerals than suggested by the official recommendations!

Portions

Never forget that you provide the quality while your child determines the quantity. This philosophy overrules any guidelines or recommendations concerning quantities.

Always remember that

- Every child has different needs;
- Every child has different likes and dislikes;
- Every child's needs vary over time;
- Every child has cravings that reflect his body's needs;
- And all this is unpredictable!

If this reality does not reassure you, you may want to rely on the tablespoon rule for security:

Feed your child one tablespoon (15 mL) of a given food for every year of life as a minimum adequate quantity, that is

- Two tablespoons (30 mL) for a two-year-old;
- Three tablespoons (45 mL) for a three-year-old;
- Four tablespoons (60 mL) for a four-year-old, and so on.

This rule applies to cooked meats, fish, poultry, liver, cottage cheese, applesauce, cooked vegetables, peanut butter, etc.

While the tablespoon rule still applies, the following chart represents the *actual* quantities of food consumed by surveyed preschoolers. The smaller intakes apply to children 18 months to three years, the larger to four- to six-year-olds. Some children demand more generous portions, which only goes to prove how complex preschoolers can be.

Actual Quantities Consumed by Preschoolers

milk	125–175 mL	$\frac{1}{2}$–$\frac{3}{4}$ cup
yogurt	50–125 mL	$\frac{1}{4}$–$\frac{1}{2}$ cup
cheese	15–30 g	$\frac{1}{2}$–1 oz.
cottage cheese	50–125 mL	$\frac{1}{4}$–$\frac{1}{2}$ cup
fish or meat	30–60 g	1–2 oz.
legumes	50–125 mL	$\frac{1}{4}$–$\frac{1}{2}$ cup
tofu	30–45 g	1–$1\frac{1}{2}$ oz.
eggs	one small	
fresh fruit	half or whole	
raw vegetables	a few pieces	
fruit juice	75–125 mL	$\frac{1}{3}$–$\frac{1}{2}$ cup
bread	half a slice to one slice	
cooked cereal	75–175 mL	$\frac{1}{3}$–$\frac{3}{4}$ cup
dry cereal	75–175 mL	$\frac{1}{3}$–$\frac{3}{4}$ cup
pasta	50–175 mL	$\frac{1}{}$–$\frac{3}{4}$ cup
rice or millet	50–125 mL	$\frac{1}{4}$–$\frac{1}{2}$ cup
butter or oil	5 mL	1 tsp.
gelatine dessert	75–125 mL	$\frac{1}{3}$–$\frac{1}{2}$ cup

Chapter Three

Instinct Versus Needs

THE ISSUE of whether or not a child will instinctively choose the right foods cannot be discussed without reviewing the classic studies done by Dr. Clara Davis in 1928.

Dr. Davis's research focused on identifying the foods that infants would select themselves in the absence of adult intervention and then tried to determine if the foods and the amounts selected were adequate to maintain growth and development. She first studied three infants, just weaned, who had never eaten solid foods. They were orphans in good health and living in a hospital. She planned their diet and observed them for a period of six to 12 months. The daily menu was built around a list of 33 highly nutritious foods that were strictly unprocessed, available fresh all year long, and served raw when possible or cooked without any added salt, sugar, or fat. Each meal consisted of one-third of the 33 foods on the list; each food was served on an individual plate. The infants were allowed to choose their own foods and determine the amounts they wanted to eat.

All three babies chose both animal and plant foods, but each ate differently. Their choices varied over time and were not predictable. Their appetites seemed irresponsible and erratic, yet they showed no sign of food intolerance and did not suffer from constipation, and they grew and developed normally.

After analyzing the results of the experiment, Dr. Davis concluded that the infants did not choose their foods by instinct but by *taste*; each child developed definite food preferences, which changed over time.

A subsequent study carried out with 12 other children fed basic, highly nutritious foods led Dr. Davis to conclude that young children's food choices *are based on their selective appetites rather than on their instincts*. The trick of the experiment was that the food list comprised natural, unprocessed, unrefined foods. Each child discovered what he liked by tasting different foods, and he could not err when only highly nutritious foods were offered.

Other studies have tried, unsuccessfully, to repeat Dr. Davis's results. When the list of foods includes processed or sweetened foods, children who select their foods cannot get the proper nourishment.

Such experiments can hardly be repeated in the home or day-care center, but two major principles remain important when planning your child's diet:

- *Always offer the most nutritious foods at every meal;*
- *Allow your child to determine the quantity he or she needs without any comments, suggestions, threats, or pressure.*

And always keep in mind that your child's seemingly erratic eating behavior is affecting *your* morale more than her development.

A recent study carried out by Leann Birch of the Child Development Laboratory at the University of Illinois reinforces the notion that children are better equipped than adults to regulate their food intake. Children who are left in control (with no external coercion) are able to regulate both the quantity and variety of the foods they eat.

In other words, if you provide the quality, you can let your child determine the quantity and you can be at peace!

As your child learns more about food, you will be learning to respect your child's inner mechanism. It is a challenge, but it is the best way to long-lasting, healthful eating habits.

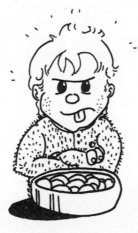

Chapter Four

The Development of Taste

WHEN A CHILD wants to eat a certain food, he really just wants to relive a happy moment experienced with that particular food.

To enjoy a food means to know it, of course!

And no doubt, whenever you offer a new food, your child says, "I don't like it; I never tried it."

Your child is continually developing a taste for certain flavors, textures, colors, and aromas. As he does so, he is slowly building special bonds with foods.

At each meal, your child increases his store of knowledge and sensations of foods. If his food memories are filled with happy sensations, he enjoys eating and stands a better chance of being well fed. Multiple happy eating experiences have a major impact on your child's sense of taste and openness to new foods.

Even though studies on the topic are far from complete, many shed new light and provide new tips on how to sell wholesome foods to your little ones.

A Taste for Chili Peppers!

How could a young child ever enjoy, even binge, on chili peppers? A study conducted in a small town in Mexico attempted to clear up this mystery. After having observed and questioned a number of families, the authors made the following observations:

- The taste for chili peppers developed gradually from the age of two to its peak at the age of eight;
- Chili peppers were introduced slowly, in very small quantities, and children were never forced to eat them. Initially, a little pepper was added to a known food, and if the child refused it, he was offered something else;
- Chili peppers were never imposed, but they had acquired the status of *adult food* in the community; the whole family, including every adult, eats them at least three times a day.

Because of this very respectful approach, the seven-year-old Mexican child ate more chili peppers than his parents, and he preferred his hot snack to a sweet or sour one!

Early and frequent exposure to a food, with no pressure other than some status building, makes quite a difference. If it can be done for chili peppers, broccoli should be a cinch.

A Taste for Vegetables

North American toddlers and preschoolers are not great vegetable lovers. The only way to "sell" unpopular vegetables is to treat your child the way you would treat your best friend:

- *Never force your child to eat* — it never works!
- *Offer small quantities*, and be a good role model;
- *Invite a friend who likes vegetables to dinner*, if your child is under four years old, he will be more easily influenced and ready to make changes than when older; he will more readily accept the influence of a child six or more months older;
- *Visit the market* to acquaint your child with vegetables in a positive way;
- *Garden or cook vegetables with your child* and have him taste just a bite; tasting has more impact than just looking;
- *Suggest tasting activities to the babysitter or day-care center;* children are quite receptive when peers are around and watching.

A Taste for Attention and Affection

Promoting healthy foods can be easier than you think!

Children respond positively to foods that are presented with warmth and affection. Making sure that meals are served in a relaxed environment is important, be it at home or at the day-care center.

A food presented as a reward stands an even better chance of being accepted. A special treat can be a carrot stick, a pepper ring, or a spoonful of sesame butter, and can achieve the same results as a cookie or candy but without the danger of tooth decay or sugar dependency!

A food lovingly offered is more likely to be associated with happy sensations than a food offered hurriedly at the counter. You can plan special occasions to introduce wholesome foods and thus positively influence your child's taste for such food.

Even in the best of circumstances, a preferred food can suddenly be refused if it is linked to an unhappy experience or a stomach upset. If you want your child to overcome such a temporary aversion, respect it regardless of what triggered it.

Changing Tastes

A child's food tastes develop in spurts. Your preschooler may be open to food adventures before the age of four, become more selective for a few years, and then become more receptive again. These fluctuations reflect the child's overall development and contribute to the shaping of his personality. Using force to impose certain foods will retard the development of taste, while using respectful and tactful strategies will broaden the range of happy food experiences. To summarize these strategies, never forget the following rules:

- *Never force your child to eat;*
- *Introduce new foods very gradually;*
- *Start with very small quantities;*
- *Use peer influence when needed;*
- *Never use pressure or bribery;*
- *Give certain foods adult-food status;*
- *Offer wholesome foods as rewards and special treats;*
- *Enjoy food with your child;*
- *Serve food with tender loving care!*

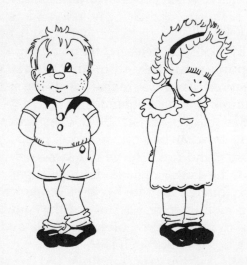

Chapter Five

Profiles of Preschoolers

EVERY SEASON in a child's life marks an important stage, and every child has his or her very own calendar of growth.

It would be impossible to describe all the possible characteristics and moods of toddlers and preschoolers since no two children are alike. However, the common features listed in the following tables can help you to better understand the eating behavior of young children from 18 months to six years of age. These tables come from two sources:

- A series of books written by two psychologists from the Gesell Institute on Child Development;
- A study conducted among 60 mothers in the Montreal and Ottawa region.

You will notice that a child's personality changes drastically from one age to another and that these modifications only last a short while. If for a given age the description does not correspond to your child at all, it may mean that your child is less excessive than average – and you can thank heaven for that! — or that she is developing at a different pace.

You can use these tables to develop the strategies, appropriate to the age of your child, that will promote happy relationships with food and improve mealtime atmosphere.

THE EIGHTEEN-MONTH-OLD

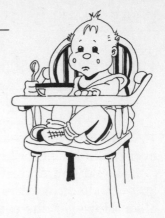

General Characteristics

- can be defined by the word "no"
- is very concerned with his property, his "mine"
- loves to go up and down the stairs
- gets into everything
- prefers to do things alone, without help
- initiates several activities in one day
- can be quite rebellious

Eating Behavior

- appetite has decreased noticeably
- agrees to be fed but will often refuse meat
- vigorously expresses preferences and dislikes
- enjoys eating when all is well
- likes to play with food
- is more skillful at drinking from a cup

Practical Suggestions

- feed your child when he is hungry even if tired
- cut food into small pieces he can place on his spoon
- decrease portions according to appetite
- respect refusals

THE TWO-YEAR-OLD

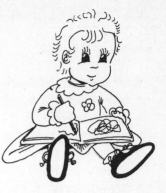

General Characteristics

- temporarily able to better express needs
- is calmer and more relaxed
- likes to store things in the same place
- loves rituals and routines
- plays alongside others
- starts to mimic

Eating Behavior

- eats alone; accepts help when tired
- is able to handle spoon
- holds a glass with one hand
- lifts glass, drinks, and puts it down
- appetite has improved somewhat
- likes to try new foods
- likes to snack between meals
- does not particularly enjoy milk

Practical Suggestions

- serve meals on a regular schedule (whenever possible)
- offer new foods when child is in a good mood
- use peer influence to ease the acceptance of a new food
- serve minisnacks
- be a good example

THE TWO-AND-A-HALF-YEAR-OLD

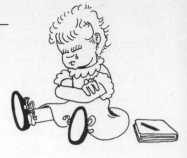

General Characteristics

- cannot make choices
- often changes mind
- insists on rituals
- feels secure on a schedule
- goes from one extreme to the other
- is quite authoritarian
- tires quickly and occasionally wants to regress
- starts playing with others

Eating Behavior

- starts to use a fork
- always asks for the same food
- loves to snack between meals
- prefers to eat from someone else's plate
- eats better in a known setting and with a known ritual
- does not particularly like meat

Practical Suggestions

- take advantage of rituals: same schedule, same place at the table, same place setting, same placemat
- use music to create a relaxing atmosphere
- do not plan too many meals outside, at a restaurant, with new friends, or in an unknown setting
- avoid bribery when faced with refusal or spontaneous strikes
- present food as a *fait accompli*, instead of asking for opinions about the menu
- give the same foods over again, if nutritious

THE THREE-YEAR-OLD

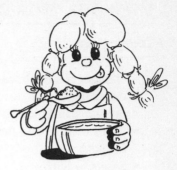

General Characteristics

- tries to please
- can ride a tricycle
- can stand on tiptoe
- likes to fingerpaint and play outside
- likes to hear stories: wants every story to be read over and over
- loves listening to music
- knows how to express wants and starts using words instead of actions
- likes to play with peers
- is less aggressive and defensive than at two and a half
- loves secrets
- is very curious

Eating Behavior

- refuses vegetables and new foods
- does not eat a lot at mealtimes
- every bite may need negotiation
- holds a spoon properly
- holds a cup by the handle with one hand
- is too small for table manners
- likes surprises: a beautiful fruit, a favorite dessert

Practical Suggestions

- avoid large servings
- never force child to finish plate
- offer new foods when child is relaxed or as a surprise
- seat near Mommy or Daddy if eating out
- pay more attention to what child eats than to manners
- keep leftovers for between-meal snack

THE FOUR-YEAR-OLD

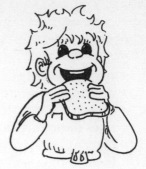

General Characteristics

- is cheerful, exuberant, full of energy, comical
- enjoys adventure, outings
- loves everything new: people, places, toys, books
- eager to learn
- rejects everything that is not "pretty"
- loves parties
- is imaginative
- can be unpredictable
- likes to negotiate

Eating Behavior

- has a better appetite than at three
- refusals and preferences are less obvious
- takes less time to eat
- still hates certain vegetables
- can pour a glass of water or milk
- drinks very quickly
- likes to set the table

Practical Suggestions

- never insist on an empty plate
- allow child to prepare meals with you
- ask child to help set the table
- let child choose new foods
- eat out once in a while

THE FIVE-YEAR-OLD

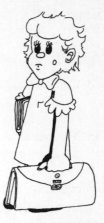

General Characteristics

- wants to please
- shows interest in room, home, street, neighbors
- has lost some of taste for adventure or new things
- is comfortable with the known
- lives in the present
- likes to finish what was started
- becomes more tense at five-and-a half

Eating Behavior

- enjoys eating certain foods over and over
- eats very slowly
- prefers simple foods and dissects complex dishes and casseroles
- does not like foods served very hot or cold
- usually finishes plate
- eats foods at restaurant refused at home

Practical Suggestions

- serve simple foods: avoid stews, gravies, sauces, or casseroles
- use outings to sell new foods
- offer lukewarm soup and allow sherbet to thaw slightly before serving
- be very patient

Chapter Six

When Your Child Refuses Foods

FOOD REFUSAL is a normal part of a child's erratic eating patterns and requires tons of patience and understanding.

Food refusals may reflect a child's insecurity and is often related to the *fear of an unknown taste*. If you present the new food as a new flavor and challenge for the tongue and if you encourage your child to just taste it with no obligation to like it or to eat it all, you may succeed in getting your child to try it.

Your child may suddenly refuse a known food that she did not really like before. Tell her that everyone has different likes and dislikes and that these likes and dislikes change over time; describe your own dislikes when you were young and explain how you came to enjoy certain foods. This relaxed approach relieves pressure and allows your child to be open to the notion that someday she may like it — she can never guess the day her taste buds will appreciate it!

Your child may refuse a food he liked before. Try to determine the reason for this change in taste. Is it a playmate's taste or a bad experience with the food in question? Ask your child why he suddenly dislikes a soup he used to enjoy so much; suggest preparing the next batch together so you can discover the faulty ingredient. It may be the carrots, which he enjoys mashed but not cut and cooked in cubes!

Your child may refuse a food in one form but love it in another. For instance he may refuse fish fillets or poultry pieces but wolf down a croquette of fish, meat, or poultry with relish! Small changes can be great solutions!

WHEN YOUR CHILD REFUSES MEAT

Preschoolers often refuse meat. Is it the texture, taste, a lack of appetite? Only the child knows. One thing is certain, your child can be healthy without eating meat every day, if he obtains adequate *protein* and *iron* from other sources.

What to Do

- Try smaller portions: 30 to 60 g (1 to 2 oz.) a day is enough;
- Serve tender, juicy meats;
- Serve ground beef in child-pleasing meatloaves and sauces;
- Serve poultry or fish instead of meat because it is easier to chew;
- Introduce cooked legumes or tofu for both protein and iron.

Why Insist on Meat?

Its high protein content helps build and repair body tissues and its iron contributes to high quality blood. However, meat is not the only source of protein and iron.

Operation Protein

These foods contain as much protein as 30 grams (1 oz.) of meat.

- 30 g (1 oz.) chicken
- 1 egg
- 125 mL ($\frac{1}{2}$ cup) yogurt
- 45 mL (3 tbsp.) cottage cheese
- 30 mL (2 tbsp.) peanut butter
- 90 mL (6 tbsp.) cooked legumes (chick peas, lentils)
- 30 g (1 oz.) cheese

Operation Iron

Regularly serve foods that are high in iron, keeping in mind that 30 grams (1 oz.) of meat contain only 1 mg of iron. The following foods contain more than that amount:

- **3 to 5 mg per portion:** liver, fortified cream of wheat, prune juice, blackstrap molasses
- **1 to 3 mg per portion:** cooked legumes, whole wheat muffins, wheat germ, oysters

The following meal plan contains no meat but provides adequate protein and iron.

SOLUTION

One Day without Meat (but with Adequate Iron and Protein)

Breakfast:	Iron (mg)	Protein (g)
125 mL (4 oz.) prune juice	5.5	0.5
1 slice whole wheat bread	0.7	3
15 mL (1 tbsp.) peanut butter	0.3	4
125 mL (4 oz.) 2% milk	0.1	4.5
Snack:		
½ bran muffin	0.7	3
Lunch:		
50 mL (¼ cup) cooked lentils	0.7	3
75 mL (⅓ cup) brown rice	0.3	1.4
50 mL (¼ cup) broccoli	0.2	1
½ apple	0.2	—
125 mL (4 oz.) 2% milk	0.1	4.5
Snack:		
125 mL (4 oz.) 2% milk	0.1	4.5
2 oatmeal cookies	2	—
Supper:		
125 mL (4 oz.) 2% milk	0.1	4.5
75 mL (⅓ cup) macaroni	0.3	1.7
30 g (1 oz.) cheddar cheese	0.7	0.6
50 mL (¼ cup) coleslaw	0.5	0.6
½ banana	0.4	0.5
	12.9	37.3

WHEN YOUR CHILD REFUSES MILK

A child may occasionally refuse milk at around 18 months or between the ages of two and three.

What to Do

- Never overreact;
- Discover the reason for the refusal: Is it the flavor, the temperature, the way the milk is served, the time of the day?
- Assess your child's current milk intake, taking into account all foods containing dairy products: 500 mL (16 oz.) of milk per day is enough to meet a preschooler's needs for calcium and vitamin D;
- Check if everyone who eats with your child drinks and likes milk.

Then

- Try serving small quantities in a "special" glass with a straw;
- If the child still refuses to drink any milk, try concealing it in soups, desserts, sauces, and shakes;
- If concealment fails, substitute other foods to fulfill the requirements for calcium and vitamin D.

Why Insist on Milk?

It is an excellent source of protein, calcium, and added vitamin D; these nutrients are essential for the growth of healthy bones and teeth.

Operation Calcium

Serve three to four times a day foods that contain as much calcium as 125 mL (4 oz.) of milk, such as

- 125 mL (4 oz.) buttermilk
- 125 mL (4 oz.) yogurt
- 175 mL (6 oz.) cream soup made with milk, fortified with 5 mL (1 tsp.) milk powder
- 30 to 45 g (1 – 1½ oz.) cheese
- 15 mL (1 tbsp.) blackstrap molasses
- 20 mL (4 tsp.) sesame butter

but avoid giving the same foods over and over.

Operation Vitamin D

Very few foods contain significant amounts of vitamin D, so it is difficult to offer as much vitamin D as in 500 mL (16 oz.) of milk on a daily basis.

Other means of getting the needed amount of vitamin is to expose your child to sunlight, 30 square centimeters (12 sq. in.) of skin, one hour per day.

If your child is not exposed to sunlight regularly, as in winter or if he never or rarely drinks milk, use a vitamin D supplement (see Appendix B, page 205).

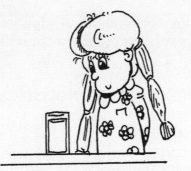

SOLUTION

Three Days without Milk (but with Adequate Calcium)

	Calcium (in mg)
Day 1: 559 mg calcium (with some dairy products)	
• 60 mL (4 tbsp.) milk powder	220
• 30 g (1 oz.) canned salmon with bones	34
• 45 g (1½ oz.) cheese	180
• 15 mL (1 tbsp.) sesame butter	125
Day 2: 500 mg calcium (with a little cheese and yogurt)	
• 50 mL (¼ cup) cottage cheese	46
• 50 mL (¼ cup) cooked broccoli	34
• 1 slice whole wheat bread	50
• 125 mL (½ cup) macaroni and cheese	208
• 125 mL (½ cup) yogurt	160
Day 3: 530 mg calcium (for strict vegetarians)	
• 50 mL (¼ cup) firm tofu* (Sunrise)	100
• 125 mL (½ cup) cooked legumes	50
• 10 mL (2 tsp.) blackstrap molasses	80
• 30 mL (2 tbsp.) dark sesame butter	200
• 45 mL (3 tbsp.) kale	50
• 45 mL (3 tbsp.) broccoli	50

* Soy milk does not provide calcium; tofu may contain calcium if prepared with a calcium-based coagulant.

WHEN YOUR CHILD REFUSES VEGETABLES

Children, especially around the age of three, often refuse vegetables. They may protest nicely or ferociously, depending on the attitudes of those around them. But with a little help, even a preschooler can be seduced by vegetables.

Choice and Presentation

- Choose vegetables that are fresh, attractive, and colorful and prepare them with care;
- Offer mini portions to start, just one or two bites;
- Offer raw vegetables rather than cooked;
- Cut vegetables into fun shapes;
- Create stories around attractive vegetables; plant a broccoli tree in mashed potatoes; present green beans or asparagus as soccer players with green peas for soccer balls.

Helpful Ideas

- Serve raw vegetables with a dip — anything sells with a dip, even raw mushrooms;
- Serve raw vegetables in fondues (see recipes);
- Serve raw vegetables in juices or fortified drinks (see recipes);
- Offer vegetables half-cooked, Chinese style, in a wok;
- Offer cooked vegetables au gratin, or with a favorite sauce or grated cheese;
- Cook vegetables in chicken or beef stock instead of water;
- Hide vegetables in soups;
- Add vegetables to a pasta recipe.

Psychosocial Strategies

- Be a good example: Eat vegetables often and enthusiastically in front of your child without ever pressuring her or commenting on her refusal to try them;
- Invite a vegetable-eater friend to dinner and serve attractive vegetables to both children;
- Use vegetables as rewards and serve them with yogurt or cheese dips;
- Promote vegetables as adult food; what is appealing to adults becomes appealing to children;

- Convince your child that she can taste the vegetable without having to like it;
- Allow your child to help prepare vegetables;
- Plant some vegetables with your child and follow their growth together.

Why Insist on Vegetables?

They are good sources of beta-carotene, vitamin C, and folic acid, as well as fiber.

Which Vegetables Are Best?

Some vegetables have more vitamins than others; if your child does not eat large quantities, give priority to the vitamin-rich ones in the following chart.

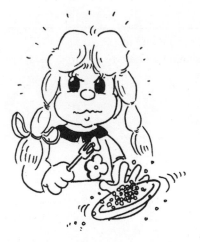

Good Sources of Nutrients*

VITAMIN A**

1122 IU	216 IU	50 IU
carrots	winter squash	green beans
spinach	tomatoes	cabbage
pumpkin	broccoli	corn
sweet potato		peas
		zucchini
		turnips
		asparagus

VITAMIN C**

30 mg	12 mg	7 mg
red peppers	cabbage	tomatoes
green peppers	spinach	peas
broccoli	turnips	asparagus
kale	cauliflower	zucchini
Brussels sprouts		potatoes

* Based on portions of 45 mL (3 tbsp.)

** For other foods containing vitamins A and C see Appendix A.

Chapter Seven

Different Diet, Different Challenge

YOUR OWN EATING STYLE will normally determine your child's diet. There are many different eating styles, or cuisines, in the world — Mexican, Chinese, French, Mediterranean — but there are only a few main diet options. These diets are defined by the food groups they contain.

The omnivorous option is a diet that includes meat, fish, poultry, eggs, dairy products, as well as all the other foods available from plant sources.

The lacto-ovo-vegetarian option is a diet that includes dairy products, eggs, whole grains and cereals, legumes, nuts, fruits, and vegetables but no meat, fish, or poultry.

The lacto-vegetarian option is similar to the lacto-ovo diet; the only difference is in the absence of eggs and egg-based products.

The strict vegetarian, or vegan, option is a diet built on plant foods exclusively. It contains no milk or eggs, or any products derived from animals, such as broth and gelatine.

The macrobiotic option is a diet based on a philosophy that aims to achieve balance between *yin* and *yang*. The menu may include some foods of animal origin, a wide variety of vegetables in season, some fruit, whole grain products, and a limited quantity of fluids, especially at mealtime.

In general, the more food groups there are in the daily diet, the less the risk of deficiencies, and the fewer the food groups on the menu, the more the risk of deficiencies. The risk of deficiencies in young children is greater because the amount of food eaten each day is somewhat limited compared with the volume eaten by an older child, a pre-adolescent, or an adult. Research carried out in recent years tends to confirm that more deficiencies are observed among vegan and macrobiotic children than among omnivorous and lacto-ovo-vegetarians. That explains why many nutrition experts do not recommend a vegan or a macrobiotic diet for children under the age of two. It is important that the diet option you adopt provides all the nutrients your child needs to grow and develop normally.

Recommended Nutrient Intakes for Preschoolers*

Nutrients	2–3 years old	4–6 years old
Calories	1300	1800
Protein	16 grams	19 grams
Vitamin A	400 ER	500 ER
	(1332 IU)	(1665 IU)
Vitamin D	200 IU	200 IU
Vitamin E	4 mg (6 IU)	5 mg (7.5 IU)
Vitamin C	20 mg	25 mg
Folic acid	50 mcg	70 mcg
Vitamin B_{12}	0.6 mcg	0.8 mcg
Thiamin	0.6 mg	0.7 mg
Riboflavin	0.7 mg	0.9 mg
Niacin	9 mg	13 mg
Calcium	550 mg	600 mg
Magnesium	50 mg	65 mg
Iron	6 mg	8 mg
Iodine	65 mcg	85 mcg
Zinc	4 mg	5 mg

Source: *Nutrition Recommendations for Canadians,* Report of the Scientific Review Committee, 1990.

* During preschool years, boys and girls have similar nutrient needs. Things change at age 7.

Diet Plan for the Omnivorous Child

This diet plan features a range of foods that complement one another and that can satisfy the nutritional needs of most toddlers and preschoolers. Supplements are required only if the child eats very little or poorly.

Milk and dairy products

- 4–6 servings a day *
- never allow more than 1 L (4 cups) of milk per day

Meat, poultry, fish, and substitutes

- 60–120 g (2–4 oz.) per day
- substitute tofu or cooked legumes a few times a week

Fruits and vegetables

- 4–5 servings a day
- serve a fruit or vegetable *high in vitamin C* at every meal to improve iron absorption
- no more than 250 mL (1 cup) of fruit juice a day

Bread and whole grain cereals

- 3–6 servings a day
- give priority to whole wheat bread or whole grain products that have no added sugar (brown rice, pasta, cereals)

---

* Serving sizes vary with age and appetite (see portion guide, page 7).

This diet plan includes dairy products and eggs, but no meat, fish, or poultry. There is no health risk if it is well planned. Supplements are required only if the child eats too little or very poorly.

Milk and dairy products

- 4–6 servings a day*
- never allow more than 1 L (4 cups) of milk per day

Protein of plant origin

- cooked legumes: 150–175 mL ($\frac{2}{3}$–$\frac{3}{4}$ cup) per day

or

- tofu: 60–90 g (2–3 oz.)
- nut or seed butter: 15–30 mL (1–2 tbsp.) a day
- bread and cereal products: 3–6 portions a day
- always give priority to whole grain products

Eggs

- 4–7 a week,
- unless there is a family history of atherosclerosis

Fruits and vegetables

- 4–5 servings a day
- serve a fruit or vegetable high in vitamin C at every meal to enhance iron absorption.
- 250 mL (1 cup) of juice a day is a maximum

---

* Serving sizes vary with age and appetite (see portion guide, page 7).

Diet Plan for a Vegan Child

This diet contains no food of animal origin and of course no dairy products. It is not usually recommended for children under the age of two because of the risk of deficiencies*. If you decide to put your child on a vegan diet, it is very important to follow the diet plan** and to give your child the appropriate supplements (see page 00).

Proteins: plant origin

- fortified soy milk***: 500 mL (2 cups) a day
- cooked legumes: 150–200 mL (²⁄₃–³⁄₄ cups) a day

or

- tofu 60–90 g (2–3 oz.) a day
- nut or seed butter: 30 mL (2 tbsp.) or more a day
- cereal products: 4–6 servings a day
- give priority to whole grain products

Fruits and vegetables

- at least 6 servings a day
- serve a fruit or vegetable high in vitamin C at every meal to enhance iron absorption

Marginal but healthy foods

- serve often because of high calcium or iron content
- 15 mL (1 tbsp.) blackstrap or green molasses
- 15 mL (1 tbsp.) dark sesame butter

---

* Some vegan or macrobiotic preschoolers have a slower growth curve than non-vegetarian children, especially before the age of two. This problem is caused by a lack of calories due to an excessive intake of fiber: Fiber-rich foods fill up a child without providing sufficient calories. Cases of rickets have been found among vegan and macrobiotic toddlers because they lack vitamin D in their diets. To prevent such problems, which can lead to permanent bone damage, provide a vitamin D supplement during winter months (see supplements chart, page 205).

** Portions vary with age and appetite (see portion chart, page 7).

*** Regular soy milk contains little calcium and no vitamin D. Fortify each 250 mL (1 cup) of soy milk with 5 mL (1 tsp.) sunflower oil, 10 mL (2 tsp.) honey or brown sugar, and 10 mL (2 tsp.) powdered calcium lactate to increase calories and calcium. Use this fortified soy milk to prepare desserts, soups, and other recipes that usually require cow's milk (see Appendix C).

Chapter Eight

Supplements

IN CANADA, 35 to 72 percent of children are regularly given a supplement of some kind, with one child in ten taking more than one supplement each day.

Do these children really need supplements? If so, are they receiving the appropriate supplement?

Some nutritionists and doctors say yes, others disagree!

Before investing in a supplement, assess your child's diet and answer the following questions:

Does my child eat
- milk and dairy products every day?
- a little meat, tofu, or legumes every day?
- some fruits and vegetables every day?
- some whole wheat bread, whole grain or enriched cereal every day?

Then assess your child's overall health and answer the following questions:

Does my child
- show normal height and weight for her age? (Your family doctor can provide you with an answer)
- have good resistance to infections?
- have a good level of energy?

If you answered yes to the previous questions, your child probably does not need any supplements.

If you answered no to one or more questions, consult Appendix A on Recommended Nutrient Intakes (RNIs) and Supplements. But before going any further, make sure you know the difference between a *multivitamin* and a *megadose*.

The Multivitamin

- Contains several vitamins;
- May contain iron and other minerals;

- Provides a dose that *rarely* exceeds five times the Recommended Nutrient Intakes (RNIs);
- Can be used to complement the nutritional intake of a child who eats very little and very poorly.

The megadose

- May contain one vitamin or several nutrients;
- Provides a dose that is 10 to 1000 times greater than the Recommended Nutrient Intakes (RNIs);
- No longer acts as a vitamin, but as a drug;
- Can have toxic effects;
- Is not recommended for young children.

Having said all this, there are circumstances where specific supplements can play a role, for instance:

- If for whatever reason your child never drinks milk or never eats other foods high in calcium (see Appendix B), consider giving a *calcium and vitamin D* supplement as a temporary or permanent measure, depending on the situation;
- If your child eats very little vegetables or fruit, consider a *multivitamin without minerals* as a temporary measure until the diet can be readjusted;
- If your child is recovering from an illness or has lost his appetite, consider a *multivitamin with iron and zinc* as a temporary measure to speed up recovery;
- If the community water supply contains little or no fluoride, add a *fluoride supplement after the age of two* to complement the content in the water and provide better protection against cavities as a permanent measure until the age of 16. The recommended dosage is 0.25 mg per day.

If in doubt, consult a professional dietitian to evaluate your child's present eating habits and to establish the best line of action.

Warning:

Some supplements can be toxic. Nearly four thousand cases of vitamin poisoning are reported each year in the United States and 80 percent of these cases involve children. So keep vitamin and mineral supplements out of reach.

Never give a child
- more than 30 mcg (1200 IU) vitamin D per day
- more than 3000 ER (10,000 IU) vitamin A per day
- more than 1 mg fluoride per day

Some supplements are coated with sugar or contain sugar. Give this type of supplement before brushing teeth.

Some supplements contain artificial flavors and food colors. If your child has allergies, identify the added substances in the supplement with the help of your pharmacist or write to the pharmaceutical company; avoid tartrazine (yellow number 5) and amaranth (red number 2) in particular.

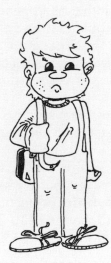

PART 2

Health Problems and
Food Remedies

"During the past several years, the scientific evidence supporting the healing power of foods has turned from a trickle into a torrent."

JEAN ROGERS,
  The Healing Foods Cookbook

Chapter Nine

Allergies

FOOD ALLERGIES are still poorly understood and remain controversial. While some experts underplay the severity of the problem, others such as Dr. Hugh Sampson of Johns Hopkins University underline the rising frequency of fatal or near-fatal food-induced reactions.

Food allergies are the body's defense mechanism against the aggression of certain foods. There are three types of reactions:

1. *An anaphylactic reaction*: symptoms appear within seconds or minutes after the offending food has been swallowed. Symptoms include a sensation of itching and tingling in the mouth, tightness in the throat, urticaria, nausea, cramping and vomiting, shortness of breath, stridor and wheezing. ***The only treatment for such a severe reaction is an injection of epinephrine within 30 minutes after the onset of symptoms;***
2. *An immediate but less severe reaction* rather like a small internal explosion that temporarily disrupts muscles, blood vessels, the skin, nose or any other part of the body. This reaction usually coincides with an evaluation of IgE antibodies in the blood;
3. *A more subtle reaction* that appears slowly after a constant intake of a particular food. Allergists then talk of a *food intolerance* or a *sensitivity* rather than a food allergy per se.

These last two types of reactions may require similar solutions, while an *anaphylactic* reaction demands ***immediate medical attention***.

Incidence

- Most food reactions occur during the first year of life;
- Most reactions are seen among children with a family history of food allergies;
- The incidence is higher and more severe among children under the age of three;
- the child most vulnerable to anaphylactic reactions has asthma and is on bronchodilating medication.

Symptoms

There is a whole range of symptoms that can be related to food allergies, intolerances, or sensitivities; the same child may exhibit more than one set of symptoms.

- *digestive problems*
    - vomiting
    - diarrhea
    - constipation
    - flatulence
    - cramps
- *skin problems*
    - rash
    - eczema
    - dark circles under the eyes
- *respiratory problems*
    - asthma
    - chronic congestion
    - chronic sore throat
- *other symptoms*
    - chronic headaches
    - muscle fatigue
    - irritability
    - behavioral problems
- *hyperactivity* can occasionally be linked to food allergies.

Before concluding that your child has a food allergy, make sure he has a thorough medical examination. Several of these symptoms can have causes other than food allergy (see also lactose intolerance, gastroenteritis, chronic diarrhea).

Foods to Watch out for

These foods are most often associated with allergies:

- milk and dairy products
- chocolate and cola
- citrus fruits
- legumes, including soybeans, peanuts, and other nuts
- corn, including corn oil and corn starch
- eggs
- tomatoes
- wheat
- cinnamon
- some food dyes, particularly tartrazine and amaranth

Beware of Botanical Relatives

- When there is an allergy to oranges, symptoms can appear with other *citrus fruits* as well: grapefruit, lemons, kumquats, tangerines, mandarines, clementines;
- The *graminae* family includes all cereals (wheat, oats, rice, millet, barley, rye) except buckwheat.

How to Detect an Allergy

Before assuming your child has a food sensitivity or allergy, try to rule out all other possible causes.

- Investigate the family's allergy history, including grandparents and first cousins: two allergic parents have a high risk of having allergic children;
- Have the child undergo a complete checkup to assess growth and weight curves, resistance to infection, current eating and sleeping patterns. Get a blood test;
- Take into account all other aspects of the child's environment, daily routine, and stresses;
- Keep a record of when symptoms occur, of suspected foods, of the frequency of occurence: Is there a reaction every time the suspected food is eaten?

Once you have done this background work, you may want to resort to allergy tests, skin, or sublingual tests (under the tongue) but you should know that these tests are unreliable for food allergies. The easiest and least expensive method is the elimination diet, but instead of eliminating single foods, you eliminate all suspected foods at once.

THE ELIMINATION DIET

1. Eliminate from the child's diet the following suspected foods for a period of ten days:
   - milk and all dairy products
   - any food containing eggs
   - any food containing gluten
   - chocolate and colas
   - foods containing food colorings, including bacon, sausages, and cold cuts (see page 105)
   - foods containing corn, including corn oil, corn flakes, corn starch, corn syrup, corn oil margarine

2. With the help of a dietitian, plan a balanced diet, taking into consideration the eliminated foods and the nutritional requirements of your child. Plan around foods that have shown low risk of allergies:

- *vegetables:* beets, spinach, broccoli, cabbage, cauliflower, turnip, Brussels sprouts, squash, lettuce, carrots, celery, sweet potatoes
- *fruits:* prunes, cherries, apricots, cranberries, blueberries, figs, papaya, avocado, rhubarb
- *meats:* chicken, turkey, lamb, rabbit, goose, game
- *cereal products:* buckwheat, rice (brown, wild, or white), bread or pasta without gluten

If the whole family can adopt this new diet, it makes it easier on the child.

3. Keep a daily record of your child's reactions as well as all the foods and beverages taken at meals or in between.

4. At the end of the ten days, begin offering one of the eliminated foods a day; note all the reactions. If the symptoms reappear, eliminate the suspected food again and then wait one or two days before giving another eliminated food.

5. If the results are inconclusive, repeat the experiment a second time, but no more.

6. If the child still has symptoms, proceed with other tests or eliminations under medical supervision.

A child suffering from food allergies may have other nonfood allergies (fur, feathers, dust) that need to be controlled before symptoms will disappear.

Long-term Treatment

A child often improves after the elimination of certain foods, but the symptoms may not always be completely suppressed. When an offending food is identified and improvement is achieved, it is important to

1. Replace the offending food by another that is equally nutritious:

- If all *dairy* products have been eliminated, the child will need an adequate supply of calcium (see page 25);
- If *eggs* are eliminated, make sure other sources of protein are included in the diet;
- If *gluten* is eliminated, try recipes with buckwheat, brown rice, or corn flour to incorporate some whole grains into the diet;
- If *corn* is eliminated, read all food labels carefully to avoid this

ingredient since it is present in many packaged foods, from corn starch to corn oil;

- If *chocolate* is eliminated, use carob to give extra flavor to cookies and drinks.

2. Plan the new diet with your child, explaining why these changes need to be made; depending on the age of your child, share the responsibilities.

3. To avoid isolating the child in his little world of allergies, adapt the new diet to the rest of the family.

4. Cook with basic ingredients to control what goes into meals; avoid ready-to-eat mixes or dishes.

5. Every six months, challenge your child with a small quantity of the problem food and observe the reactions. If the child reacts well, gradually reintegrate the food; if not, drop it for another six months. If the symptoms are severe, these periodic challenges should be done by a doctor to avoid any possibility of anaphylactic reaction.

Difficult Occasions

If you want to make it easier for your child to respect his food allergies, you need to think out all situations where food will be offered, for example:

Day-care center: Provide the caregiver with a complete list of problem foods including brand names of processed foods that contain the offending ingredient; submit a list of suggested menus and recipes that could be offered to all children periodically; offer to bring along a batch of muffins or cookies that are good for everyone.

Birthday parties: Advise the host not to embarrass your child in front of the others and to provide him, if necessary, with his own piece of nonchocolate cake and candies without food colorings. If your child is faced with a series of forbidden foods, a nice strategy is to promise him a reward when he goes back home so that the word *party* continues to mean a special occasion!

Eating out: Check restaurant menus ahead of time to make sure the chosen restaurant has foods the child can eat, and remember that it is better to stay home than have an outing turn into a source of tears and frustration.

Easter and chocolate: Find another super-surprise for the whole family to smoothly eliminate the association of holiday and chocolate.

Picnics: Give your child extra allowed foods so that he can share his food with the others and not feel left out.

PROBLEM

Normal Diet

Breakfast:
orange juice
wheat cereal with milk
½ slice *toast*
2% milk

Snack:
cheese cubes

SOLUTION

Elimination Diet

Day 1

white grape juice
Granola Special with
    soy or **Almond Milk**
½ banana

raw vegetables (carrots, green
pepper, celery) and tofu dip

SOLUTION

Day 2

Buckwheat Pancake
Spring Compote
soy or **Almond Milk**

Banana Almond Muffin

Lunch:		
egg sandwich	tomato juice	**Lentil and Apple Soup**
raw *vegetables*	tuna and rice salad	rice biscuit
Jell-O	**Fresh Fruit Jelly**	raw vegetable salad
2% milk	soy or **Almond Milk**	grape juice jelly
Snack:		
chocolate chip cookie	½ banana	½ pear
Supper:		
chicken *pâté*	grilled or roasted chicken	**Shrimp Paella**
small green salad, dressing with *corn* oil	baked potato	small broccoli or cauliflower salad
upside down *cake* with apples	coleslaw with sunflower oil dressing	**Carob Cake**
2% milk	applesauce	soy or **Almond Milk**
	soy or **Almond Milk**	
Snack:		
fruit-flavored drink		

Foods in *italics*: source of problem
Foods in **bold**: recipes included in this book

Chapter Ten

Anemia

WHILE THERE ARE FOUR different types of anemia that can affect children, *iron-deficiency anemia* is the type seen most frequently among preschoolers and is the one that will be discussed here.

There is a high risk of iron deficiency during any intense growth period since new tissues of the body and the brain require more iron to develop and function properly. About 70 percent of the iron in the body is in the form of hemoglobin, which transports and distributes oxygen to all body cells.

Iron-deficiency anemia is indicated by a lower level of hemoglobin in the blood. An iron deficiency not only affects the quality of the blood but, because it slows down the transportation of oxygen, can alter other functions such as a child's learning capacity and his general attitude toward his environment. It can jeopardize a child's mental and physical development.

Incidence

The problem is common among preschoolers in both industrialized and developing countries; in Canada, the diets of nearly one child in two under the age of five are iron deficient.

Increased Vulnerability

The most vulnerable period is between the age of six months and three years, beginning when iron stores present at birth are depleted until the child begins to eat enough of a variety of iron-rich foods. Premature children and those with low birth weights are more vulnerable than full-term and adequate-birth-weight babies. The next most vulnerable period is during adolescence.

Symptoms

- chronic fatigue, pallor, loss of appetite
- low weight gain, irritability
- concave instead of convex nails
- very red, sore tongue
- compulsive consumption of ice or other nonfood substances

- lack of interest in the outside world
- decreased learning capacity

To check if these symptoms are truly caused by an iron deficiency, the doctor may recommend a blood test to measure hemoglobin levels and the degree of saturation of the transferrin.

Causes

The major cause is a *lack of iron* in the diet. Since a child's iron stores are precarious, iron must be obtained from food sources. An adult can recycle 95 percent of the body's iron while a child only recycles 70 percent.

Other causes are poor iron absorption, caused by faulty food combinations at mealtime, and excessive milk intake, which decreases the child's appetite for iron-rich foods and competes for proper absorption.

Treatment

To eliminate symptoms and replenish the child's iron stores, the family doctor will usually prescribe an iron supplement in the form of *ferrous sulfate*; this supplement is given in the morning and at bedtime since it is best absorbed on an empty stomach. To avoid staining the teeth, place the supplement on the back of the tongue before swallowing.

Most symptoms will disappear within a few days, but it may take a few months to replenish the depleted iron; that is why you must continue giving the supplement for one or two months after the normal level of hemoglobin has been reached.

In the meantime, gradually improve the child's diet, and offer several iron-rich foods daily (see the ABCs of Prevention).

Side Effects of Iron Supplements

Although rare, some children experience gastrointestinal problems. Caution! Iron supplements are the second largest cause of accidental poisoning among young children after Aspirin; keep the supplements out of reach!

The ABCs of Prevention

Iron deficiency anemia is relatively easy to prevent; as soon as you introduce solid foods, always include iron-rich foods in your child's diet (see page 49).

Since the second year of life is the most vulnerable, keep *iron-fortified infant cereal* on the menu; serve plain, mixed with mashed carrots or applesauce, or add to cream soups, yogurt, or other desserts.

Once or twice a week, serve a superdish made with liver or kidneys; very fresh calf's liver is quite tasty.

- Serve puréed chick peas, lentils, white beans, and other legumes in soups or dips or try a lentil spaghetti sauce;
- Offer whole wheat bread instead of white bread;
- Add dried fruits, wheat germ, carob, wheat bran to muffins and breads;
- Prepare fruit jellied dessert with iron-rich prune juice;
- Limit milk intake to 750 mL (24 oz.) a day;
- Avoid foods that are low in iron such as candies or soft drinks.

To increase iron absorption, serve a fruit or vegetable rich in vitamin C at every meal (see page 00).

Foods That Increase Iron Absorption

- Even a small quantity (30 g/1 oz.) of meat, fish, or poultry will increase the absorption of iron contained in vegetables and cereal products;
- Fruits and vegetables rich in vitamin C make a big difference.

Foods That Inhibit Iron Absorption

- Tea
- Excessive amounts of milk and dairy products
- Antacids and certain antibiotics

 PROBLEM

 SOLUTION

Diet Low in Iron	Iron (mg)	Diet Rich in Iron	Iron (mg)
Breakfast:			
orange drink	—	½ grapefruit	0.5
2% milk (250 mL/1 cup)	—	fortified cream of wheat (75 mL/⅓ cup)	5.2
½ slice toasted white bread with jam	0.3	2% milk (200 mL/6 oz.)	—
Snack:			
glass of milk	—	celery stick	0.2
Lunch:			
chicken noodle soup (125 mL/½ cup)	0.3	**Lentil Soup** (125 mL/½ cup)	2.5
½ slice white bread	0.3	carrot sticks	0.5
cheese (30 g/1 oz.)	0.2	½ slice whole wheat bread	0.4
strawberry Jell-O	—	small orange	0.4
2% milk (250 mL/1 cup)	—	2% milk (124 mL/4 oz.)	—
Snack:			
glass of milk	—	½ pear	0.2
Supper:			
shepherd's pie	2.1	**Small Fortified Pâtés**	9
small slice of cake	0.3	½ baked potato with skin	0.4
2% milk (250 mL/1 cup)	—	broccoli florets	0.4
		applesauce	0.6
		2% milk (175 mL/6 oz.)	—
	3.5		20.3

Foods in **bold**: recipes included in this book.

Preschooler's iron needs: 6–8 mg per day.

Chapter Eleven

Atherosclerosis

THE NORTH AMERICAN CHILD *has one chance in three of developing a cardiovascular problem before he turns 60. Atherosclerosis kills more Canadians each year than any other disease, but statistics show a decline in deaths from cardiovascular problems since the early 1970s.*

This is the reality. However, there are no grounds for cholesterol phobia, but there is room for a better understanding of the issue as it relates to the preschooler.

Atherosclerosis usually develops silently over at least 40 years before problems show up, often in the form of a heart attack. Fatty substances adhere to the lining of the arteries and the build-up eventually prevents normal blood flow.

Family history and lifestyle can both lead to a coronary disaster. Researchers have even noticed that members of the same family (parents, siblings) seem to have similar blood cholesterol levels as long as they live together, but when they stop living under the same roof, the trend changes.

The Vulnerable Child

Vulnerability merely indicates a higher risk level and should be considered a prediction only. The vulnerable child has one or more parents or grandparents who have had a heart attack or a high blood cholesterol level before the age of 50. The child may also live in a family of smokers, eat a high fat diet, and do little physical activity.

How the Problem Develops

The blood and blood vessel lining change over the years and tend to reflect lifestyles and family history. In a vulnerable child, the progression may be as follows:

- By age ten, fatty streaks start appearing in the arteries;
- By 20 years of age, fibrous plaques begin to narrow the arteries;
- At around 40, especially in men, the plaque hardens and thickens and finally obstructs the flow of blood through the arteries, causing a cardiac accident; in women this outcome is usually delayed until after menopause.

The ABCs of Prevention

Evidence strongly suggests that the benefits of reducing blood cholesterol in childhood will be realized in adulthood, while no study has yet been able to demonstrate the advantages of an excessive intake of cholesterol, saturated or hydrogenated fats, sugar, calories, cigarettes, or a lack of exercise!

The prevention strategy is not specifically aimed at lowering the child's blood cholesterol level but at promoting good living and eating habits. It is easier to learn how to eat and live healthfully at three or four than to convert at 40!

The best strategy is the *family approach* and involves everyone in the child's immediate environment: grandparents, baby-sitters, day-care staff. The attitudes and behavior of those surrounding a child have much more impact than all the nutrition lectures in the world.

Prevention includes:

1. *An annual medical checkup* to track the
    - Growth curve;
    - Blood pressure after the age of three;
    - Blood cholesterol level if the family history suggests it (a parent has had a heart attack before 55 or a high blood cholesterol).

2. *A balanced diet,* including a moderate intake of essential fatty acids (see chart) and adequate protein and fiber. There is no need to eliminate saturated fats and cholesterol: From the age of two through adolescence, there should be a gradual transition from the high-fat diet of infancy to an adult diet that includes no more than 30 percent of calories as fats and no more than 10 percent of calories as *saturated* fats.
3. *Physical exercise,* with the family or with other children; encourage activities that can be practiced at any age, such as walking, dancing, skating, or riding a bicycle.
4. *A smoke-free environment.* Avoid smoking in the home. It is never too early to start a subtle anti-tobacco campaign: smokers are three times more likely to develop cardiovascular problems, especially if they start smoking before the age of 20.

Foods That Contain Essential Fatty Acids

- sunflower, corn, safflower, sesame, or soya oils
- olive and canola oils

- sunflower seeds, almonds
- salmon, sardines, mackerel, trout

Foods High in Saturated and Hydrogenated Fats

- butter, lard, shortening
- margarines*
- beef, lamb, pork, cold cuts, goose, duck, mutton
- cheese made with whole milk
- coconut and palm oils
- chocolate, cocoa powder, coconut
- cream substitutes containing coconut or palm oils
- egg yolk
- pastries made with the above ingredients
- whole milk, yogurt made with whole milk
- crackers*, cookies*, chips*
- regular peanut butter*

* high in hydrogenated fat

On the other hand, if the child has a high blood cholesterol level, he must follow a more rigorous diet to control his condition and prevent future problems.

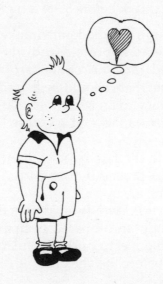

PROBLEM

Diet High in Fat

	Fat (g)
Breakfast:	
orange in sections	—
egg, boiled	6
toasted bread with margarine	10
whole milk (250 mL/8 oz.)	9
Lunch:	
carrot sticks	—
minipizza with ham and cheddar	17
banana	—
whole milk (250 mL/8 oz.)	9
Supper:	
vegetable juice	—
ground beef (90 g/3 oz.)	17
potato with butter	5
broccoli with butter	5
custard	5
whole milk (250 mL/8 oz.)	9
	92

SOLUTION

Diet Moderate in Fat

	Fat (g)
orange in sections	—
whole grain cereal with	
2% milk (125 mL/4 oz)	3
Bran Muffin	4
2% milk (250 mL/8 oz.)	5
carrot sticks	—
minipizza with 2% cheese	10
Miracle Compote with Sesame Seeds	5
2% milk (250 mL/8 oz.)	5
vegetable juice	—
baked filet of sole (90 g/3 oz.)	1
with lemon juice and olive oil	5
baked potato with yogurt and chives	—
steamed broccoli	—
strawberry jellied dessert	—
2% milk (250 mL/8 oz.)	5
	43

Foods in **bold**: recipes included in this book

Chapter Twelve

Constipation

CONSTIPATION IS A PROBLEM of infrequent, painful bowel movements or hard, dry stools.

The condition varies greatly from one child to another. Some experts consider it to be a form of body language, used to express silent emotions, while others see it as the result of a low-fiber diet, inadequate fluid intake, or poor toilet training.

Normally foods that are not absorbed continue through the large bowel and are slowly pushed toward the rectum by a series of contractions. After each meal or snack, there are stronger contractions, and when a certain food volume reaches the rectum, the pressure triggers the need to go to the bathroom, especially 15 to 30 minutes after breakfast.

When a child ignores the message, the food stays in the lower part of the large bowel; this waste-removal system becomes less and less responsive. Once the lower part of the bowel becomes accustomed to retaining the additional load, it stops sending the message to defecate. Part of the water contained in the stool returns to the upper bowel, stools become harder and drier, and elimination becomes difficult and painful; the vicious cycle of constipation has begun.

Incidence

The problem is quite common among preschool children.

It is seen more often in boys than in girls and more often among hyperactive children.

Impact on Health

Stagnating food waste in the bowel is not toxic, but the pressure it exerts on the rectum may cause headaches, irritability, and discomfort. In other words, constipation can make a child's life miserable.

Acute Constipation

Acute constipation occurs when the bowel suddenly stops functioning. This interruption can happen when a child changes diet or environment, decreases her physical activity, is on a trip, or is sick.

Although rare, it can be caused by an anal fissure. Things usually return to normal once the child goes back on her routine.

Regular Constipation

The problem of chronic hard, dry stools is seen more often before the age of four. Among possible causes are the fear of pain, a diet low in fiber, a lack of physical activity, insufficient fluids but a large milk intake (more than one liter a day), the wrong position during defecation, and poorly established bowel habits. Treatment includes

- Establishing a regular toilet schedule;
- Increasing fiber intake;
- Limiting the daily consumption of milk (750 mL/24 oz.) and cheese;
- Using 2% milk instead of whole milk;
- Increasing physical activity.

Make sure your child's feet touch the floor or other support when at the toilet to help the contractions.

Try not to make a big fuss over the issue!

Chronic Constipation

This problem is serious and relates to irregular defecation, painful elimination, and occasional soiling; it is more common after the age of four. This *pain-retention-pain* cycle is often the complication of untreated regular or mild constipation.

Among possible causes are emotional problems, tension or anxiety, fear of going to the *school* bathroom, and poor toilet training.

Treatment requires time and patience and a global approach. Initially, you may need to resort to drastic measures (enema, laxatives). To loosen stools, use 15mL (1 tbsp.) of *mineral oil* a day for a couple of months; this amount will not cause any vitamin deficiency.

- Increase the fiber intake; begin by adding a daily tablespoon of natural wheat bran in yogurt or applesauce; consult the sample menu on page 58 to add more fiber-rich foods on a daily basis;
- Insist on a good breakfast;
- Plan an extra 15 to 30 minutes after meals to wait for the natural impulse;
- Increase fluid intake, especially water, at mealtime and in between;

- Gradually stop laxatives and carefully note the frequ
  defecations.

Success may be long term if you maintain the new habits!

The ABCs of Prevention

When your child is around two years old, establish a good toilet-training routine and develop a relaxed attitude about it.

- Offer foods that are rich in dietary fiber at every meal;
- Encourage your child to chew all foods well;
- Never skip breakfast;
- Promote physical activity;
- Serve meals on a regular schedule, whenever possible.

Enemas and Laxatives

These are temporary solutions to use only when a blockage is serious.

Fiber Ideas

- Offer whole wheat, bran, or rye breads instead of white bread;
- Serve bran cereal (All-Bran, Bran Flakes, Raisin Bran, Bran Buds and Psyllium) instead of refined cereal;
- Serve raw vegetables and small salads instead of juice or cooked vegetables;
- Serve whole fruits instead of fruit juices.

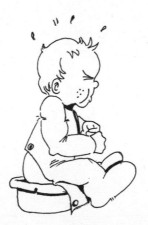

PROBLEM

Diet Low in Fiber

	Fiber (g)
Breakfast:	
orange juice	—
refined cereal (75 mL/$\frac{1}{3}$ cup)	0.3
2% milk (175 mL/6 oz.)	—
Snack:	
slices of cucumber, peeled	—
Lunch:	
chicken noodle soup	—
$\frac{1}{2}$ cheese sandwich on white bread	—
strawberry Jell-O	—
2% milk (175 mL/6 oz.)	—
Snack:	
chocolate chip cookie	—
Supper	
green salad	0.4
ground beef with mashed potato	1.5
small cooked carrots	1.7
ice cream	—
2% milk (175 mL/6 oz.)	—
	3.9

SOLUTION

Diet High in Fiber

	Fiber (g)
2 cooked prunes	1.3
All-Bran cereal	3.1
2% milk (175 mL/6 oz.)	—
3 carrot sticks	1.3
Lentil and Apple Soup	2.3
1 slice whole wheat bread	2.6
½ apple	2.0
2% milk (175 mL/6 oz.)	—
small bran muffin	2.7
carrot and raisin salad	1.9
Meat Loaf in Disguise	2.5
cooked broccoli (50 mL/¼ cup)	1.4
orange sections	1.2
2% milk (175 mL/6 oz.)	—
	22.3

Foods in **bold**: recipes included in this book

Chapter Thirteen

Diarrhea

CHRONIC DIARRHEA, also called *chronic nonspecific diarrhea* (CNSD), is a problem of frequent, liquid stools that can last a few days or up to a few months without any other disquieting symptoms. There maybe four to six watery stools a day. The condition is sometimes called the *irritable colon syndrome*, or the green peas and carrots syndrome, since these vegetables are easier to trace in the stools.

Chronic diarrhea should not be confused with the soft stools that result from a wholesome high-fiber diet, with lactose intolerance accompanied by bloating and cramps, or with malabsorption problems such as celiac disease.

Possible Causes

Chronic diarrhea can be a side effect of diet restrictions maintained long after an episode of gastroenteritis or any other infection. It can result from excessive fluid intake (more than $1\frac{1}{2}$ L (6 cups) a day); sensitive children cannot cope with such an overload of fluids.

A *low-fat diet* perpetuates the problem while substituting milk with large quantities of juices, sweetened fruit-flavored drinks or soft drinks increases the quantity of poorly digested carbohydrates and aggravates the problem.

A large intake of foods containing fructose and/or sorbitol, prunes, pears, peaches, apple juice, cola drinks, figs, and dates often creates the problem. Children under five actually drink 36 liters (9 gallons) of juice a year, of which 50 percent is apple juice!

Stress caused by an infection can also temporarily prevent the proper functioning of the digestive system.

Incidence

The problem usually appears after a change of diet due to an infection. It is more frequent between six and 30 months and in boys.

Most toddlers outgrow the problem by the age of four or five.

How to Know When It Is Serious

- If your child is pretty resistant to infections and maintains his growth curve, you do not need to worry;
- If your child's growth chart shows a decrease in the rate of weight gain, there may be a malabsorption problem and you should seek medical advice.

Suggested Treatment

Proceed one step at a time:

- Start by going over your child's diet with a dietitian to identify any possible problems;
- Reduce fluid intake to a maximum of $1\frac{1}{2}$ L (6 cups) per day, half in the form of milk and most of the rest in water;
- Eliminate fruit juices that are rich in sorbitol and fructose: prune, pear, sweet cherry, peach, apple juices. Instead, serve *diluted* orange or pineapple juice in small quantities to a maximum of 175mL (6 oz.) a day;
- If there is no improvement after a week, increase your child's fat intake to 50 grams a day to slow down the elimination process.
  - Serve whole milk instead of partially skimmed milk;
  - Add a little butter or homemade dressing on vegetables;
  - Serve cheese and peanut butter more often.

When everything is back to normal, gradually return to a leaner diet.

The ABCs of Prevention

- Resume a varied diet as soon as possible after an episode of gastroenteritis or any other problem;
- Limit fruit juice to 175 mL (6 oz.) a day, and choose juices that contain less fructose and sorbitol (pineapple, orange);
- Limit total fluid intake to a maximum of $1\frac{1}{2}$ L (6 cups);
- Maintain an adequate fiber intake.

SOLUTION

Recovery Diet to Eliminate Chronic Diarrhea*

Breakfast:
half an orange in sections
whole wheat toast with butter and peanut butter
175 mL (6 oz.) whole milk at room temperature

Snack:
a small cube of cheddar cheese

Lunch:
half a whole wheat pita bread stuffed
    with eggs and mayonnaise
carrot sticks
applesauce
175 mL (6 oz.) whole milk at room temperature

Snack:
half a slice of toast with peanut butter

Supper:
60 g (2 oz.) ground beef or salmon
half a potato, with a little butter
green beans
half a banana with vanilla yogurt
175 mL (6 oz.) whole milk at room temperature

---

*Quantities may vary according to the child's age and appetite.

Chapter Fourteen

Gastroenteritis*

GASTROENTERITIS is also called *acute diarrhea* or the *flu*. It is a very serious problem. It begins with sudden diarrhea, nausea, and vomiting; fever follows in 50 percent of cases. This infectious disease causes major loss of water and minerals that are essential for the proper functioning of the child's body. The rapid dehydration can be quite damaging

Incidence

Nearly 500 million children under five years of age are affected each year throughout the world, more frequently in winter than in summer. Acute diarrhea is one of the most common infections in North America; it leads to dehydration, which causes 500 deaths per year in the United States among preschoolers. Most of these deaths could be prevented by *proper fluid replacement*.

Possible Causes

Gastroenteritis is caused by a virus in four out of five cases. In certain areas of the country, contaminated water may be another cause.

When to Consult Your Doctor

If your child passes three or more liquid stools in a day, vomits, and is exceptionally thirsty, consult your doctor as soon as possible; young children are particularly vulnerable.

The ABCs of Home Treatment

As soon as the symptoms are identified, start rehydrating your child with the recommended fluids: provide approximately 125 to 175 mL (4 to 6 oz.) of fluids *per hour* if your child weighs 10 kg (22 lb.) and up to 150 to 275 mL (5 to 9 oz.) *per hour* if your child weighs 15 kg (32 lb.). Offer the liquid at room temperature, 15 to 30 mL (1 to 2 tbsp.) at a time, every 10 to 15 minutes. If your child drinks sufficiently, he will recover more rapidly and regain his appetite faster.

---

*See also chronic diarrhea.

As soon as your child regains his appetite, give him foods that he likes and can digest easily, and gradually add all the elements of a balanced menu (meat, fruit, vegetables, cereal products); reintroduce milk five to seven days after the beginning of the illness.

Fasting Is Not Recommended

Fasting is not recommended: This traditional cure prolongs diarrhea instead of curing it. After a few days without food, the child is weak at a time when she must rebuild energy and resistance. Fasting deprives her of the nutrients essential to recovery.

Recommended Fluids

Many, many fluids have been recommended throughout the years, from cola to Jell-O to chicken bouillon. The proper fluids can rehydrate your child more rapidly and replenish lost nutrients.

The ideal fluid contains the same proportions of glucose, sodium chloride, and potassium as the child's body fluids; that way the fluid is better absorbed and the body will retain all the nutrients that can shorten the duration of the disease:

- *Breast milk* is recommended for unweaned babies;
- *Certain commercial drinks* (Gastrolyte, Lytren, Resol, Infatyle) available in drug stores can be used for the first 24 hours;
- A *homemade drink* can also be given as long as all the ingredients are measured accurately:

    1 L (32 oz.) tap or spring water
    2 mL (½ tsp.) salt
    1 L (32 oz.) unsweetened orange juice from frozen
    concentrate, diluted as usual
  Stir very well and keep refrigerated. Stir before serving.

The proper fluids will not stop the diarrhea instantly, but they will replace the water and minerals lost through diarrhea and vomiting and prevent dehydration.

Drinks That Do Not Really Help

- Tap water or bottled spring water is not absorbed by the digestive tract; it goes straight through;
- Undiluted fruit juices provide an excessive amount of sugar and lack the sodium required for absorption;
- Soft drinks, Jell-O, and Popsicles are too sweet and lack

potassium, while tea, rice, and barley water are altogether too low in sugar, sodium, and potassium;

- Cow's milk, whole or skim, is temporarily difficult to digest because of a short-term lactose intolerance.

Such drinks are better than nothing, but they do not promote recovery.

What to Do Next

- If your child does not react positively to the rehydration treatment in the first hours consult your doctor again;
- *If your child has very dry skin and cries without tears, he is seriously dehydrated and needs to be hospitalized immediately;*
- If your child succeeds in drinking regularly and eating solid foods with appetite, there is no need to worry even if the stools remain abnormal for one or two weeks.

Gastroenteritis Is Contagious

Gastroenteritis is an infectious disease that spreads easily. Other members of the family should stay away from the sick child and avoid eating from the same plates.

Points to Remember

Do not wait for your child's stools to get back to normal before feeding solid and varied foods. If your child is drinking fluids every hour, is not vomiting anymore, and is hungry, start feeding her as soon as she wants to eat.

It is important that you provide foods that compensate for losses, but serve small amounts of each food at first to facilitate absorption. Give priority to favorite and easily digested foods.

SOLUTION

Recovery Diet for Gastroenteritis*

Breakfast:
cream of wheat
applesauce
orange juice (diluted 50-50)

Snack:
orange juice (diluted)
half a slice of toast

Lunch:
soft-boiled egg
cooked carrots
toast
small ripe banana
orange juice (diluted)

Snack:
orange juice (diluted)
applesauce

Supper:
chicken and cooked vegetables
steamed or boiled rice
fruit jellied dessert
fruit juice (diluted)

---

* It is important to reintroduce all the basic foods including milk one week after the beginning of the illness.

Chapter Fifteen

Hyperactivity

HYPERACTIVITY is now called *Attention Deficit Disorder* (ADD) or *Attention Deficit Hyperactivity Disorder* (ADHD).

This condition has attracted media attention for the past 20 years, but it still is not fully understood by modern medicine because of the vast range of symptoms and possible causes. Diagnosis is difficult since no lab test exists that can confirm or negate the condition.

The American Psychiatry Association defines ADD as inappropriate inattention, impulsivity, and hyperactivity for a given mental and chronological age. It corresponds to superactive behavior but not to an intellectual deficit or a brain disfunction.

The problem should be constant and noticed by more than one adult in the child's environment for at least six months before a parent should start worrying and searching for a solution.

Incidence

Researchers estimate that three to five school-age children out of one hundred may be affected to various degrees. The problem is seen three to eight times more frequently in boys than in girls, and has been observed around the world, in both rural and urban areas.

Common Symptoms

Symptoms are not usually noticed during the first 24 months but become more obvious and specific between the ages of two and six. It is often difficult to differentiate ADD from normal disruptive behavior.

Around the age of two, people might say this child

- Never walks but always runs;
- Climbs over everything;
- Changes activity every ten seconds;
- Never stops;
- Does not like to be cuddled.

Around the age of three or four, people might say this child

- Is demanding and disruptive;
- Never listens;
- Has difficulties playing alone or with others;
- Is unable to concentrate;
- Does not react to rewards or punishment;
- Reacts to the first signs of rejection by friends;
- Has difficulties with passive activities;
- Cannot finish what he starts;
- Does not tolerate any frustration;
- Sleeps poorly.

Causes

Causes remain a puzzle, but there may be a genetic component and a family history of allergies. Among other possible causes:

- Lead poisoning, which can be detected with a blood test;
- An intolerance to sugar (see page 71);
- Allergy or hypersensitivity to certain foods like chocolate, wheat, and corn (see page 39);
- Lack of essential fatty acids, characterized by constant thirst;
- Psychosocial factors.

Until now, the hypothesis that has attracted most attention was developed in the seventies by Dr. Ben Feingold and relates hyperactivity to food allergies, including hypersensitivity to food colorings and artificial flavors, to certain additives, and to salicylates in aspirin and in some fruits and vegetables.

If your child displays the symptoms of Attention Deficit Disorder for at least six months, your family doctor should investigate all possible causes — medical, social, and environmental, including an analysis of the child's daily activities.

Treatment

1. Minor changes in the child's environment can reduce stimuli and increase self-esteem: giving the child more attention, serving a favorite healthy snack, inviting a best friend over to reinforce an improved behavior.
2. An improved diet can do no harm!

    Dr. Feingold's K-P diet resulted in improvement in 5 to 10 percent of children who reacted favorably to the elimination of all sources of salicylates, food colors, and artificial flavors as well as food additives. The reason why Dr. Feingold's diet does not always work is that it proposes the *same diet for all children* regardless of the cause of the hyperactivity; it requires no nutritional evaluation, provides no replacement for a missing nutrient, and does not eliminate other possible sources of food allergy. To improve the Feingold method, a study was done at the Alberta Children's Hospital with 24 hyperactive preschool boys using a more personalized diet planned after an evaluation of each child's nutritional status; the core of the diet contained a very limited amount of sugar but no artificial colors and flavors, chocolate, monosodium glutamate, preservatives, or caffeine and eliminated any other suspected food. The results showed improvement in behavior among half the group, which is far better than just 5 to 10 percent.

Long-term adherence to such a program has shown continued behavior improvement for most children.

If your child has had a complete medical examination and still has

- problems sleeping
- cramps and chronic diarrhea
- a constantly runny nose
- frequent headaches
- sugar cravings
- reactions to certain medications
- reactions to certain foods
- and frequent food refusals

you have nothing to lose by getting an evaluation of your child's nutritional status and by following an elimination diet for seven to ten days (see page 66) to check for any possible food allergy or intolerance. You can then restructure the diet for the whole family accordingly; if you include nutrient-dense foods, you will improve the overall nutritional quality of the menu.

3. Use a vitamin or mineral *supplement*, if needed, but not a *megavitamin* (large dosage of some vitamins) — such large doses have been used without success and pose potential danger.
4. If your hyperactive child is always thirsty, use a supplement of essential fatty acids, available in the form of evening primrose oil over-the-counter in drugstores and health food stores.
5. Behavioral therapy.
6. Family therapy.

7. Medication prescribed by your doctor should be the last resort. The usual medications (dextroamphetamine, methylplenidate, or pemoline) have an immediate effect on the child's attention span but may cause loss of appetite, initial weight loss, and a reduction in growth. To reduce these side effects, give medication just before or with meals and discontinue during summer months to promote catch-up growth. Monitor growth every six months.

Most of these strategies are quite demanding but they can help you make a difference.

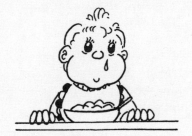

Chapter Sixteen

Hypoglycemia

HYPOGLYCEMIA HAS HAD MEDIA COVERAGE but little medical attention because it may be linked to several causes that are difficult to identify; the abnormal drop in blood sugar levels can vary from one child to another and triggers a range of behavioral problems.

Organic hypoglycemia is a symptom of an organic problem such as a tumor of the pancreas, a deficiency of certain enzymes necessary to process sugar, or a liver disease. Such conditions are very rare in young children.

Reactive hypoglycemia may be related to a diet high in refined sugar and foods and low in dietary fiber leading to an excessive production of insulin followed by low blood sugar levels.

Ketotic or *idiopathic hypoglycemia* is the most common form of childhood hypoglycemia. It typically occurs after a longer than usual fast or during an illness. It is sometimes described as the Sunday morning fit and happens when the parents sleep in and the child misses breakfast.

Diagnosis

Ketotic hypoglycemia (the Sunday morning fit) can be detected by *elevated serum ketones* in the blood during a hypoglycemic episode or after a 16-hour fast.

Reactive hypoglycemia can be detected before the age of five by measuring the blood glucose level during a spontaneous behavior change or energy drop.

Incidence

Ketotic hypoglycemia does not occur frequently but peaks at around 18 months; it is most often seen in *underweight* preschool children who are picky eaters.

Reactive hypoglycemia is seen most frequently in school children and adolescents with poor eating habits.

Symptoms

Reactive hypoglycemia can be suspected in three-, four-, or five-year-olds if

1. The child has a series of benign, unspecific problems that resemble those of hyperactivity (see page 67) or symptoms more specific to a hypoglycemic child such as

   - Extremes of behavior — sometimes quiet, sometimes agitated;
   - Unstable energy;
   - Unpredictable episodes of spontaneous sleep;
   - Abnormal fatigue considering the amount of sleep obtained.

2. The child has very poor eating habits:

   - Almost never eats breakfast;
   - Drinks fruit drinks and juices all day long;
   - Goes many hours without eating a real meal;
   - Has sugar binges;
   - Eats mainly refined foods: white bread, rice, pasta, and cookies.

Dietary Intervention

When your child's symptoms and diet suggest *reactive hypoglycemia*, you should attempt a change in diet for one or two months.

The new diet is quite simple and essentially improves the quality and distribution of foods throughout the day. The purpose is to stabilize the blood sugar levels by avoiding all foods that can increase it abruptly. You should do the following:

- Feed your child more often and more regularly;
- Include three small meals and three to four small snacks;
- Eliminate or reduce to a minimum all *sugar* intake, white sugar, brown sugar, honey, molasses, jams, maple syrup, as well as any foods containing sugar (see page 115);
- Substitute refined products with whole grain products:
  - offer whole wheat bread instead of white bread
  - bake with whole wheat flour instead of white flour
  - serve brown rice instead of white rice
  - serve whole wheat noodles instead of white flour noodles; they are easy to find and so tasty!
  - serve unsweetened oatmeal instead of refined and sweetened cereals

- Eliminate fruit-flavored drinks and soft drinks, as well as fruit juices, since these foods are quickly absorbed and can raise blood sugar levels too rapidly;
- Serve raw and cooked vegetables, as well as fresh fruit more often;
- Plan sugar-free snacks that contain protein and fiber: milk, yogurt, toast with peanut butter, cheese cubes, and pieces of fresh fruit.

If symptoms vanish or decrease substantially during this dietary intervention, maintain this new diet.

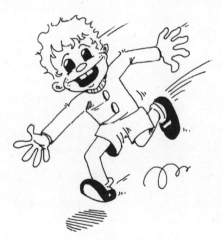

 PROBLEM

 SOLUTION

Diet High in Sugar and Refined Foods	Diet without Added Sugar, High in Dietary Fiber
Breakfast:	
fruit drink	orange sections
white toast	oatmeal with finely chopped
jam	almonds
	milk
Snack:	
cola or fruit juice	raw vegetables with cheese or peanut butter
Lunch:	
chicken noodle soup	raw vegetables
salted crackers	half a sandwich with cheese and
chocolate chip cookies	salmon on whole wheat bread
fruit drink	with alfalfa sprouts
	pineapple slice in its own juice
	milk
Snack:	
chocolate chip cookies	plain yogurt
Snack:	
cola or fruit drink	
Supper:	
hot dog	brown rice with chicken
fries	broccoli or Brussels sprouts
chocolate milk	fresh **Fruit Kabob**
	milk
Snack:	
fruit drink	whole wheat muffin

Foods in **bold**: recipes included in this book.

Chapter Seventeen

Lactose Intolerance

LACTOSE INTOLERANCE IS THE INABILITY to digest the *lactose* in milk and other dairy products. It is not a *milk allergy* (see page 39).

Lactose, the natural sugar in milk, is usually digested in the small bowel with the help of *lactase*, an enzyme produced in the brush border of the bowel. When lactase is deficient, lactose enters undigested into the large bowel, where it ferments and causes discomfort. Absorption still takes place but in a painful way.

The symptoms range from abdominal pains, cramps, colic, and gas to diarrhea, 30 minutes to three hours after drinking milk or eating other lactose-rich foods. The severity of these symptoms varies with the individual and with the quantity of lactose consumed.

Incidence

The world is divided in two: *lactose digesters* and *lactose nondigesters*. Lactose digesters include descendants of Northern Europeans, the Fulani and Tussi tribes of Africa, the Punjabi of India, Finns, and Hungarians. The rest of the world's peoples are lactose nondigesters. This group includes Asian, Native American, Mexican, Inuit, and Arab children and adults.

Over the years the intermixing of races has increased the number of *lactose digesters*; for example, Black and Native Americans have become progressively better able to cope with lactose.

The problem seldom occurs in preschool years and among white children, but there are always exceptions.

When the condition appears suddenly after an illness, and lasts for a few weeks, it is called a temporary intolerance. If it lasts longer, the term *prolonged intolerance* is used.

Foods Containing Lactose

- Whole milk, partially skimmed or skim milk, yogurt, buttermilk, sour cream, table and whipped cream, whole or skim milk powder;
- Foods prepared with milk powder such as breads, rolls, muffins, cakes, or cookies;

- Foods prepared with milk such as soups, sauces, and puddings;
- Homemade or commercial mixes to which milk or powdered milk has been added;
- Ice cream and sherbets, chocolate and sweets prepared with milk;
- Certain margarines containing milk powder;
- Some cheeses: cottage cheese, ricotta, and other nonfermented cheeses. Other cheeses such as cheddar, Edam, Swiss cheese, Camembert, and brick contain little or no lactose.

Always read labels to verify the presence of milk or other lactose sources.

Temporary Intolerance

There may be a *temporary intolerance* when the lining of the small bowel has been seriously upset and cannot produce enough *lactase*, the digestive enzyme. A temporary intolerance manifests itself by liquid stools, cramps, and other abdominal discomforts and can happen

- During gastroenteritis;
- While on antibiotics;
- After surgery of the digestive tube.

Suggested Treatment

A temporary intolerance normally disappears within a week or two, once the bowel lining is healed.

A small quantity of milk (125 to 175 mL/4 to 6 oz.) or yogurt taken at meals will usually cause less problems than large quantities (more than 175mL/6 oz.) taken between meals. Plain yogurt or cheddar-type cheeses are better tolerated than liquid milk.

Never wait more than 10 to 15 days to reintroduce the whole range of milk products.

Prolonged Intolerance

- The problem increases with age in vulnerable children: Asian, African, Mexican, and Native;
- Even small quantities of milk are enough to trigger symptoms in some children; use other foods or supplements to make up for a possible lack of calcium.

Suggested Treatment

1. Establish your child's tolerance level: give a small quantity of milk (about 175 mL/6 oz.) during a meal and observe the reaction:
   - If the child suffers no abdominal pain, colic, bloating, or diarrhea in the following hours, it means that he can tolerate this quantity *within a meal*;
   - If, on the contrary, the child suffers discomfort in the following hours, decrease the quantity of milk and observe once more;
   - If the symptoms are present even with a smaller quantity of milk given at meals, try adding a few drops of a commercial yeast-based enzyme (Lactaid) to a liter (quart) of milk 24 hours before serving.

   Lactase activity is protected by the presence of lactose, so it is better to keep a small quantity of milk in the diet than to eliminate it completely.

2. Make sure your child receives enough calcium and vitamin D. Add other rich sources of calcium to the diet (see Appendix A).

Appropriate Test

Before making any major change in your child's diet, your family doctor may recommend the *hydrogen breath test*, a painless procedure that measures the hydrogen expired in the child's breath after a large quantity of lactose. The test should take place over a period of three hours to detect the intolerance.

Lactaid (the enzyme)

Lactaid is the name of a yeast-based commercial enzyme that behaves like lactase and relieves discomfort in intolerant children, allowing them to drink milk. It does not affect the flavor of the milk and is sold over-the-counter in drugstores or health food stores. You simply add four or five drops per liter (quart) of milk and let rest in the refrigerator 24 hours before serving. Certain studies prove that it is possible to use the enzyme at the last minute: in this case add four to five drops for every glass of milk just before drinking. This latter method is efficient but more expensive.

Lactaid or Lacteeze (the milk)

You can now buy in food stores across the country milk already treated with the commercial enzyme. This milk, called Lactaid or Lacteeze, is partially skimmed at 2 percent and can be served without any drops and digested without any cramps.

 **PROBLEM**

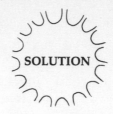 **SOLUTION**

Diet High in Lactose*	**Diet Low in Lactose****
Breakfast:	
orange in sections	orange in sections
cereal with *milk*	whole wheat toast
milk (175 mL/6 oz.)	peanut and *sesame butters*
	milk (100 mL/3 oz.) or Lactaid or Lacteeze milk (175 mL/6 oz.)
Snack:	
milk drink (175 mL/6 oz.)	raw vegetables
Lunch:	
creamed vegetable	coleslaw and **broccoli**
half a chicken sandwich	half a sandwich with **canned salmon**
caramel *pudding*	*yogurt* (125 mL/4 oz.)
Snack:	
chocolate *ice cream*	frozen banana
Supper:	
vegetable juice	vegetable juice
meat loaf	grilled meat
carrot rings	carrot rings
whole wheat bread	whole wheat bread
yogurt	fruit jelly and **sesame square**
milk (175 mL/6 oz.)	milk (100 mL/3 oz.) or Lactaid or Lacteeze milk (175 mL/6 oz.)

* Although not unhealthy, this diet is hard to digest for a child suffering from lactose intolerance.

This menu proposes foods other than milk that are rich in calcium (in **bold italics); it can also contain varying quantities of milk and yogurt according to your child's tolerance level.

Foods in *italics* contain milk or milk powder.

Chapter Eighteen

Obesity

AS EARLY AS THREE years old, a child begins to have a negative perception of obesity. Please do not reinforce this negative feeling even if you have to deal with the problem.

Obesity is an excess of *fat* not just an excess of *weight*: a child can be heavy for his age without necessarily having too much fat.

The problem is more difficult to assess in a young child than in an adult: weight is only a warning; measuring skinfold thickness (fat under the skin in the triceps area) confirms the degree of fatness.

Childhood obesity is a growing problem in North America; it affects 27 percent of children and 21 percent of adolescents in the United States. At a workshop sponsored by the National Institute of Child Health and Human Development, researchers concluded that in the last 20 years obesity has increased 54 percent among six- to 11-year-olds. A research team recently found that most children who are obese at age seven became obese at age four. *Preschool years are critical in the development of lifelong obesity*. The most important medical consequence of obesity in the young is the 70 percent risk of its persisting into adulthood.

Most of the information on obesity and its cures scratches the surface of the problem. It promotes false hopes and offers false remedies; the current obsession with thinness creates more problems than does the plumpness of a toddler. Reports of serious growth retardation in children aged nine to 17 show that some North American children do not eat enough food for fear of obesity.

Some Facts

- Breast-feeding and the *slow* introduction of solids are two excellent practices during the first year of life, but they don't guarantee lifelong thinness;
- Most chubby newborns or six-month-old babies do not become obese adults;
- A normal weight two-year-old is not protected against obesity for the rest of her life;
- Multiplication of fat cells during the first two years of life does not necessarily determine the future weight of an individual;

- There can be as many periods of fat-cell multiplication as durable weight changes during a lifetime. If you lose weight and keep it off, you lose a certain number of fat cells, and conversely, if you put on weight and maintain it, you gain new fat cells;
- A fat or overweight child does not necessarily eat more calories than the slim or normal weight child, but she eats beyond her own needs;
- It is very difficult to predict the future weight of a chubby-cheeked toddler. A weight problem is not irreversible if it is caught in time and treated properly.

A good relationship with the right foods is built long before your child learns how to read!

Possible Causes:

Heredity and environment are possible causes. Supporters of the heredity theory state that a child has a 70 percent chance of becoming obese if both parents are obese and a 40 percent chance if only one parent is affected. Supporters of the environment theory claim that an adopted child or a child living in a foster home will quickly reach the same level of overweight as her adoptive parents. But the following are also contributing factors:

- a lack of physical activity
- emotional overeating
- an overdose of television viewing
- indulgence
- neglect

Feeding a child for the wrong reasons can lead to a distorted relationship with food and promote overconsumption. Soothing a child with a candy, amusing her with a cookie, or punishing her by denying dessert will slowly encourage a poor relationship with foods. So many adults use food to solve other problems.

Complications

Short-term complications include:

- low self-esteem
- rejection by peers
- low physical performance
- loneliness
- poor relationship with foods

- loss of pleasure in eating
- stressful meals associated with reprimands and restrictions

Long-term complications include:

- higher incidence of hypertension
- higher incidence of asthma
- higher incidence of diabetes
- cardiovascular problems
- profound discomfort with food.
- skill deficits that preclude involvement in sports, dance, etc.

The ABCs of Prevention

If a child has overweight or obese parents, prevention should start from the very first years of life. In order to be effective, changes should be made by the *entire* family. The prevention strategy is based on three major, equally important components:

1. *A positive attitude toward prevention:*

- Preparing leaner meals is as much fun as cooking super-rich and more conventional recipes;
- Never associate words such as diet or sacrifice with this new way of eating;
- Adapt special occasion meals to the leaner guidelines to avoid giving your child double messages;
- Offer occasional treats without expressing remorse or referring to them as cheating;
- Avoid talking about weight and calories day after day, meal after meal.

2. *Paying special attention to the quality of the foods eaten by the entire family or those eaten with the child:*

- Give priority to basic foods such as milk, poultry, fish, vegetables, whole grain products, fruits;
- Promote foods that are rich in dietary fiber (raw fruits and vegetables, cereals, and whole grain breads);
- Serve fruit for dessert instead of rich, sweet pastries, cakes, and cookies;
- Limit juices and fruit-flavored drinks; did you know that three glasses of juice provide 360 calories — as many as five slices of bread!
- Serve this leaner menu to the whole family to promote long-lasting good eating habits for your child.

3. *A major effort to increase the family's physical activity:*

- Draw up a plan for regular physical exercise and make it a family practice; it is more fun to burn calories than to cut them!
- Take a walk every evening after supper;
- Plan outings for the whole family: walks in the country, skating, or swimming;
- Develop the physical potential of your child by getting her involved in at least one sport that is suited to her likes and abilities;
- Adopt a dog and have your child take it for regular walks or suggest that your child walk the neighbor's dog, for lack of his own!

These measures will help everyone in the family to lose a few pounds and develop a better relationship with food and exercise.

Policy makers should initiate other measures, such as those presented to President Bill Clinton in 1993 (see Appendix D), to combat the situation.

Treatment

If your three- or four-year-old has gained more than $2\frac{1}{2}$ kg (5 lbs.) during the last year while the medical checkup is otherwise normal *do not overreact*, but do take the matter seriously while there is still time!

Try to *decrease your child's rate of weight gain* by improving his diet and increasing his regular physical activity. Do not attempt to trigger a major weight loss because that can affect the child's overall development. For example, if a four-year-old gains $7\frac{1}{2}$ kg (15 lbs.) in one year (what most children gain in three years), the goal will be to allow her to grow while maintaining her weight until she is six or until her weight is suitable for her height.

To achieve this decrease in the rate of weight gain, you should provide a better choice of foods and improve your attitude toward food, and make it a family matter! A child who is put on a diet, who must follow a special set of restrictions and yet sees the rest of the family eating forbidden foods will most likely develop a poor relationship with himself and with food and become forever trapped in the vicious circle of diets.

Initially, you should

- Assess the past year to gain a better understanding of the reasons for the weight gain. The loss of a friend; the mother's going back to work; a new day-care center, environment, or routine; an illness that resulted in less physical activity and loss of appetite can all be the cause. Start a food diary and record *everything* the child eats and drinks, at and between meals, during a regular week;

- Compare your child's intake with the minimum quantities (page 7) and note any excesses;
- With the help of a dietitian, readjust the diet and replace some calorie-dense foods with fiber-rich foods that are low in fats and sugar.

Some Suggestions for Substitutions

- Serve partially skimmed milk instead of whole milk (but not until the age of 12 months);
- Serve fresh fruit instead of fruit juices or fruit-flavored drinks, or even better, offer water between meals instead of juices or drinks;
- Offer whole wheat bread without butter instead of white bread with butter or margarine;
- Serve unsweetened whole grain cereal instead of refined and sweetened cereal;
- Serve fish and poultry more often and beef less often; avoid sausages, pâtés and other cold cuts;
- Serve baked or boiled potatoes instead of fries;
- Offer frozen yogurt instead of ice cream;
- Serve foods plain or with lean sauces made with puréed vegetables, puréed fruits, or skim milk.

Good Habits to Instill

- Organize the child's eating routine so that he eats three meals a day and, if needed, one or two snacks;
- Use nonfood items to reward good behavior: a new story instead of a cookie, a game instead of a candy;
- Avoid empty plate contests. Praise your child if she leaves a little food to share with the birds or the dog;
- Adopt a new eating pace so that the fun lasts longer. Foods eaten in a hurry do not really nourish!
- Promote meals without distractions, without television, so that your child can really benefit from his food;
- Cultivate a positive attitude toward nutritious and light foods. Never label them as foods we-have-to-eat-in-order-to-lose-weight; offer them as fun foods to discover and enjoy;
- Plan a program of physical activity.

SOLUTION

Prevention Diet for Obesity

DAY 1

Breakfast:
1 orange in sections
muesli
milk 2%, 1%, or skim

Snack:
celery sticks

Lunch:
Lentil and Apple Soup
muffin with wheat germ
small salad with grated carrots
    and yogurt dressing
peach
milk 2%, 1%, or skim

DAY 2

fresh or frozen strawberries
    without sugar
Homemade Granola
milk 2%, 1%, or skim

pepper rings

vegetable juice
macaroni with cottage cheese
small coleslaw
plain yogurt with pineapple
milk 2%, 1%, or skim

DAY 3

half a pink grapefruit
cream of wheat with prunes
milk 2%, 1%, or skim

carrot sticks

small celery salad
sandwich with tofu and tuna
pear stuffed with strawberries
milk 2%, 1%, or skim

Snack:
half an apple with a
little peanut butter

1 clementine or half a banana

apple rings

Supper:

tomato juice
Fettuccine with Vegetables
small spinach salad
applesauce
milk 2%, 1%, or skim

tomato juice
Salmon Soufflé
broccoli
whole wheat bread
Peach and Prune Jelly
milk 2%, 1%, or skim

tomato juice
Chicken Almondine
small lettuce salad
vanilla yogurt
milk 2%, 1%, or skim

Foods in **bold**: recipes included in this book.

Calorie-saving Suggestions

	Savings	
By serving daily	Daily	Weekly
skim milk instead of whole milk 525 mL (18 oz.)	138	966
skim milk instead of 2% 525 mL (18 oz.)	62	411
low-fat Mozzarella instead of cheddar cheese 30 g (1 oz.)	42	294
plain yogurt instead of fruit-flavored yogurt 125 mL (4 oz.)	50	350
1 fresh pear instead of 2 halves canned pears in syrup	56	392
1 fresh peach instead of 2 halves canned peaches in syrup	80	560
$\frac{1}{2}$ plain baked potato instead of $\frac{1}{2}$ baked potato with 5 mL (1 tsp.) butter	35	245
unsweetened applesauce 125 mL (4 oz.) instead of $\frac{1}{8}$ apple pie	252	1764

1 slice whole wheat bread without butter
   instead of 1 slice whole wheat bread with
   7 mL ($\frac{1}{2}$ tbsp.) butter
	51	357

1 slice banana bread instead of banana cake with icing (1 piece)	253	1648
baked fish instead of lean beef roast 60 g (2 oz.)	143	1001
chicken burger 60 g (2 oz.) chicken, $\frac{1}{2}$ bun) instead of a hamburger (60 g (2 oz.), $\frac{1}{2}$ bun)	29	203

* The calorie savings chart demonstrates how easy it is to modify the diet; it does not imply that you should be counting the calories in every food! Counting calories is useless.

Chapter Nineteen

Tooth Decay

TOOTH DECAY, a problem common to 98 percent of the population, is relatively easy to prevent, or at least minimize.

Tooth decay is a sure sign of the destruction of the tooth, starting with the enamel and going toward the root. This condition can cause infections, speech problems, or chewing problems, and many hours of pain; it can lead to the extraction of a temporary tooth and possibly impair the proper positioning of permanent teeth.

Incidence

- At three or four years, 40 to 55 percent of children already have one cavity;
- At 12, children have an average of five cavities;
- By age 17, 94 percent of children and adolescents have had caries in their permanent teeth;
- We see less cavities than 20 years ago among school-age children but surprisingly more among preschoolers.

Periods of Increased Vulnerability

- Between four and eight years we observe cavities in temporary teeth;
- Between 11 and 18, cavities occur among teenagers;
- Between 55 and 65, the roots decay.

Normal Development of Teeth

The first set of teeth as well as the permanent teeth are in place under the gums well before they appear in the mouth; they are the product of a long underground activity. Starting during the prenatal period until the age of eight, minerals join together and crystalize inside the gums to form teeth and await eruption; the first, or baby, teeth develop until about the age of two, and permanent teeth until the age of 13.

Then, in a second round of events, the tooth emerges through the gums and the new enamel becomes vulnerable to the environment.

Several nutrients such as protein, vitamins A and C, calcium, phosphorus, vitamin D, and fluoride work from the inside during childhood and early adolescence to contribute to the formation of good permanent teeth.

Cavities

The mouth normally contains bacteria, which can be eliminated with a good brushing. If this is neglected, the bacteria multiply and cover the teeth with a thin, transparent, sticky film called *plaque*.

Plaque works like a filter; it allows sugar to pass through and change into acid; this acid then attacks the enamel, allowing bacteria inside the tooth, thus promoting the development of cavities.

Causes of Tooth Decay

Experts agree that there are multiple causes, involving more than just foods; including the following:

- *Sweet foods* remain the foremost cause, but caries have declined in recent years, although total sugar consumption has remained constant;
- *Poor dental hygiene*: inadequate or irregular brushing;
- *Weak tooth enamel*;
- *Ineffective saliva*.

Problem Foods and Medications

- Candy, refined sugars, jams, and jellies;
- Other foods naturally high in sugars such as dried fruits, honey, molasses, maple syrup, and many others;
- Cookies, breads, cakes, soft drinks, and other sweetened beverages consumed between meals;
- Cough syrups and other liquid medications containing sugar (see Appendix B, page 205) that have to be taken a few times a day or at bedtime.

The ABCs of Prevention

Good prevention includes regular visits to the dentist. Choose a friendly dentist and plan the very first visit as a social one, when your child is about three years old, so that he gets used to the chair, the environment, and opening his mouth!

Teeth Brushing

When she first begins to brush, your child will need help, then a lot of coaching and encouragement.

Brushing ideally should take place after every meal, or a minimum of twice a day; you can store a tooth brush in the snackbox that she takes to the day-care center.

Toothpaste

Toothpaste is not essential, but it can improve the resistance of the tooth if it contains fluoride. The flavor also promotes longer brushing.

Fluoride

Fluoride teams up with other minerals in the initial construction of the tooth; it inhibits mineral losses and contributes to the formation of a stronger enamel, more resistant to cavities. It seems to be able to repair partially decalcified enamel.

If applied topically, fluoride disturbs the work of the bacteria and slows down the formation of plaque.

Fluoridated Water or Supplements

Both fluoridated water and supplements are efficient and comparable. Supplements should be taken regularly up to 13 or 14 years, if local water contains no fluoride. Both methods can reduce cavities by up to 60 percent.

Recommended Quantities

If water is not fluoridated, give 0.25 mg fluoride to chidren over the age of two.

Dental Floss

- You may start flossing once a day at age three;
- Your child will need help to do a good flossing until the age of eight.

Vaccine Against Tooth Decay

Studies conducted in England foresee the eventual use of a vaccine that would be effective for at least two years. "However," says one of the inventors, "people will have to keep on brushing their teeth since this vaccine is not effective against root cavities or plaque, which is responsible for gum inflammation."

The ABCs of Prevention

Prevention involves promoting the development of healthy teeth with a diet containing adequate protein, vitamins C, A, and D, calcium, phosphorus, and fluoride, from conception throughout childhood.

Prevention includes limiting the consumption of sweet foods and drinks, especially between meals. Offer sugar-free snacks instead (see list below).

You need to establish, and supervise, a brushing and flossing routine at least twice a day; make it a game so that it becomes fun, not just an obligation.

If the community water supply is not fluoridated, give a daily fluoride supplement, or a weekly sodium fluoride solution, or plan regular topical applications.

Serve foods that are high in dietary fiber such as fresh fruits and raw vegetables because they increase the production of saliva and insure better natural cleansing action in the mouth.

Some Sugar-free Snacks

- cheese cubes or yogurt
- fresh fruits (apples, pears, oranges, peaches, bananas, melons)
- raw vegetables (carrots, celery, peppers)
- homemade rusks
- peanut butter on whole wheat bread
- vegetable juice
- whole grain cereal with milk

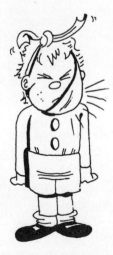

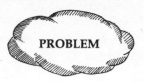 

PROBLEM   SOLUTION

Preventing Tooth Decay

DIET HIGH IN SUGAR	DIET LOWER IN SUGAR

Breakfast:
orange juice
white toast with jam
chocolate milk

orange sections
whole wheat toast with cheese and
   applesauce
2% milk

Snack:
candies

raw vegetables

Lunch:
SpinachQuiche
white bread
green salad with dressing
chocolate pudding
chocolate milk

Spinach Quiche
whole wheat bread
green salad with dressing
peach jelly
2% plain milk

Snack:
chocolate chip cookie
fruit-flavored drink

pieces of apple with peanut butter

Supper:
Salmon Croquettes
rice
broccoli
cake with caramel sauce
chocolate milk

Salmon Croquettes
rice
broccoli
Apple and Almond Custard
2% plain milk

medication containing sugar
given at bedtime before brushing
teeth

Foods in **bold**: recipes included in this book

RAMPANT TOOTH DECAY

Rampant tooth decay is a contagious form of tooth decay that affects all the superior front teeth (also called the *nursing-bottle syndrome*). It is a painful condition that can lead to speech impairments, require costly treatment, and even disfigure a child.

Incidence

At most risk are children that go to sleep with a bottle containing milk, sweetened water, juice, or any drink other than water; it usually occurs between the ages of 12 and 48 months. Also at risk are children who suck lollipops all afternoon or who use a bottle of fruit juice as a pacifier.

Cause

The bedtime bottle, pacifiers dipped in syrup, and any other sweet liquid are the prime causes.

When the child falls asleep, some of the sweet liquid stays in his mouth and the flow of saliva decreases; instead of neutralizing the mouth's environment, the sweet liquid (containing some form of sugar — milk lactose, sucrose, glucose, fructose) promotes the formation of acid, which attacks the enamel while the child sleeps.

The ABCs of Prevention

The American Academy of Pediatrics strongly recommends that all babies be offered a cup by nine months and be completely weaned from the bottle by 12 months:

- Never offer a bottle at bedtime;
- Never offer a pacifier that has been dipped in a sweet liquid, whatever it may be.

PART 3

Food Facts and Fallacies

"Consumers are bombarded with information about nutrition, some of it scientifically sound, but much of it half-true, misleading or downright false."

ELEANOR WILLIAMS AND MARY ALICE CLIENDO
  Nutrition

"It has become obvious that our food supply is undergoing an extremely rapid change, from primary foods to highly processed convenience foods. Our ability to manipulate the composition of these foods to improve the health of the consumers has hardly been used."

JEAN MAYER
  Human Nutrition

Chapter Twenty

Microwaves, Barbecues, and Pressure Cookers

USING A MICROWAVE OVEN

Foods cooked in a microwave oven are not radioactive, nor are the containers in which the foods are cooked. However, 483 young children were treated for burns caused by microwaves in 1988 in the United States. A *Good Housekeeping* survey showed that 65 percent of children under the age of 12 use microwave ovens, many of them without proper instruction.

What Is Microwave Cooking All About?

Microwaves emit radiation somewhere between radio waves and infrared rays:

- These waves can easily penetrate foods that contain water;
- Once in the food, the waves make the water molecules move, which stimulates the quick production of heat throughout the food;
- The more water a food contains, the quicker it is heated; a vegetable heats up much faster than a piece of meat of the same size and weight;
- These waves cannot penetrate metals; they bounce off, which explains why foods cannot be properly cooked in metal containers; in fact, microwaves can even damage the oven when they bounce off metal or foil;
- Microwaves penetrate glass and plastic and can properly heat foods placed in glass, ceramic, or porcelain containers and on certain papers.

The Impact of Microwaves on the Nutritional Value of Foods

- Foods cooked or heated in a microwave oven usually retain as much or even more vitamins and minerals than when cooked in a traditional manner;
- Vegetables microwaved with a minimum quantity of water retain more vitamin C than when boiled in water on the stove; the vitamin retention is similar to steaming or cooking with very little water;

- Research concerning other food components has been minimal, and the overall impact of microwaves on food is still to be studied.

- Follow the manufacturer's instructions for use and safety measures;
- Never use the oven if the door does not close perfectly, if the oven is damaged during transportation, or if there are other problems;
- Never touch the oven's security lock or controls to stop it while functioning;
- Never insert any object around the security seal;
- Clean the door and the seal regularly according to the maker's instructions and don't use abrasive substances;
- Contact the distributor if you are concerned about any problems, and have the oven checked by a competent person.

FOODS COOKED ON THE BARBECUE

A meal cooked in the garden or a park is a happening! The smell of burning wood or coals and the excitement of eating tasty foods outdoors make for special meals. However, a high-fat, *carbonized* food can be a health hazard to adults as well as preschoolers.

Two-year-olds will not enjoy this kind of meal as much as a three-year-old or an older child.

What Happens to Barbecued Foods?

- When you cook high-fat meat a few inches over burning charcoal, the fat drips into the fire and becomes benzopyrene (a carcinogenic), which then unites with the smoke and returns to the meat;
- A 120 g (4 oz.) charcoal broiled steak contains as much benzopyrene as the smoke from 135 cigarettes!

To Have the Fun without the Benzopyrene

- Use a minimum number of coals to prepare the fire: 30 to 40 coals for a big barbecue, and 12 to 24 for a Hibachi;
- Let the coals burn 30 to 40 minutes before starting to cook; coals are ready when covered with grey dust;

- Trim *all* excess fat from meat;
- Choose leaner foods such as poultry or fish more often than red meat;
- Cook foods in foil for part or all of the cooking time;
- Cook 10 to 12 cm (5 to 6 in.) away from coals to avoid intense heat.

Meals to Barbecue

I. Small cabbage and carrot salad
   Tuna and Cheese Burger
   Grilled Apple on a Stick

II. **Corn on the Cob *en Papillotte***
    Stuffed Pita Bread
    Popsicle with fruit juice and yogurt

III. **Carrots *en Papillotte***
     Fish Kabob
     Cheesy Potato
     Slice of cantaloupe with strawberry purée

IV. Raw vegetables
    Grilled Cheese
    Fruit Kabob

Foods in **bold**: recipes included in this book.

FOODS COOKED IN A PRESSURE COOKER

Foods that are cooked very rapidly in a small amount of water retain more vitamins and minerals than foods cooked for a longer time in a lot of water. A pressure cooker cooks foods quickly, using a very small quantity of water and considerable pressure.

- Foods cooked in a pressure cooker will retain more vitamins and minerals than if cooked in 125 mL ($\frac{1}{2}$ cup) of water (see chart);
- Steaming or microwaving will have similar results to cooking in the pressure cooker;
- The water added to the pressure cooker or used for steaming will collect a certain quantity of vitamins and minerals; keep it to cook rice or other cereal, or for soups and sauces.

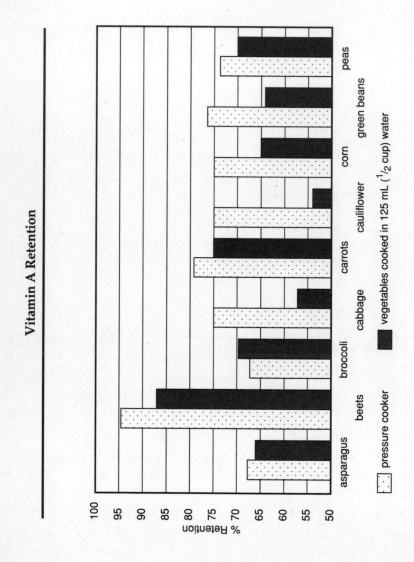

Vitamin A Retention

% Retention

100 95 90 85 80 75 70 65 60 55 50

asparagus beets broccoli cabbage carrots cauliflower corn green beans peas

☐ pressure cooker

■ vegetables cooked in 125 mL (¹/₂ cup) water

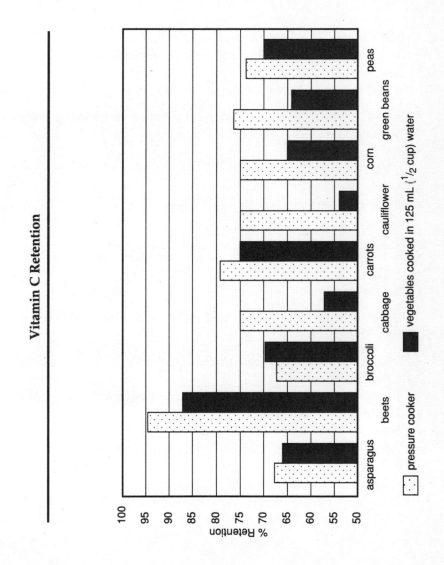

Vitamin C Retention

% Retention

asparagus beets broccoli cabbage carrots cauliflower corn green beans peas

▨ pressure cooker

■ vegetables cooked in 125 mL ($^1/_2$ cup) water

Chapter Twenty One

Fast Foods

FAST-FOOD OUTLETS attract thousands of children and adults; in Canada alone the industry has sales of more than four billion dollars per year.

As a rule fast foods provide the following:

- Excessive fats and salt in most main dishes (see tables on pages 101 and 102);
- Few vegetables;
- Few fresh fruits;
- No whole grain products;
- Very little vitamin C, calcium, or fiber.

Their success lies in other factors:

- Food is served quickly, great for the impatient young child;
- Food is usually easy to handle;
- The environment does not call for refined table manners.

If your child eats this type of food on a regular basis, it is important to improve his choices.

- Help him choose vegetable or fruit juices instead of soft drinks or fruit-flavored drinks;
- Choose plain milk instead of the ultra-sweetened milk shake;
- Choose grilled foods over fried;
- Choose a restaurant with a salad bar;
- Choose small portions, whenever possible;
- Find a quiet spot and take time to eat slowly;
- Vary the diet by alternating restaurants;
- If necessary, bring your own raw vegetables, a fruit, or milk from home to complete the menu.

Hidden Fats in Fast Foods

1 pat of butter or margarine = 4 grams of fat = ■
½ pat of butter or margarine = 2 grams of fat = ◢

homemade grilled burger   ■ ■ ■
Big Mac   ■ ■ ■ ■ ■ ■ ■ ■ ■

baked potato   —
small portion of fries   ■ ■ ◢

filet of fish, baked   —
Filet-O-Fish   ■ ■ ■ ■ ■ ■ ◢

250 mL (1 cup) 2% milk   ■
milk shake   ■ ■ ■

125 mL (½ cup) ice cream   ■ ■
banana split   ■ ■ ■ ■

apple   —
apple turnover   ■ ■ ■ ◢

boiled egg   ■ ◢
Egg McMuffin   ■ ■ ■ ◢

125 mL (½ cup) boiled onions   —
125 mL (½ cup) fried onions   ■ ■ ■ ■

Italics indicate fast foods.

Hidden Salt in Fast Foods

FOOD	SODIUM (mg)
90 g (3 oz.) grilled chicken	74
90 g (3 oz.) *fried chicken*	275
6 *Chicken McNuggets*	487
homemade hamburger without salt	158
hamburger	418
homemade fish burger	225
Filet-O-Fish	811
boiled egg with 2 slices toast	333
Egg McMuffin	806
fresh apple	2
apple turnover	326
300 mL (10 oz.) partially skimmed milk	155
chocolate milk shake	263

Italics indicate fast foods.

Chapter Twenty-Two

Canned Foods

NEVER KEEP FOODS in an open can. Store leftovers in a nonmetal container.

Lead Poisoning

- Fifty percent of the lead in your child's environment comes from foods, canned foods in particular; the rest comes from contaminated air and water;
- A study conducted in the United States a few years ago revealed that one child in 18 suffered from lead poisoning and that the most vulnerable children were between two and three years old;
- A young child absorbs three to five times more lead than an adult, who eliminates it more easily;
- Lead poisoning affects mainly the nervous system, and it can modify a child's behavior and intellectual abilities;
- In Canada, some manufacturers have eliminated the use of lead for welding cans on a voluntary basis. Imported canned foods from less-industrialized countries still pose a risk but Health and Welfare do regular checks to detect high lead levels in imported cans. When the can is opened, the air reacts with acid foods such as tomatoes, fruits, and fruit juices and dissolves part of the lead, which then gradually contaminates the food;
- A malnourished child who does not eat enough calcium-rich and iron-rich foods is more vulnerable to lead poisoning than a well-fed child;
- While the lead content in cans has decreased over the last 15 years because of improved manufacturing methods, it is still essential to remove the food from the can once opened;
- A severely malnourished child who gradually develops behavior problems should have a blood analysis to check lead levels.

Salt and Sugar in Canned Foods

- Canned fish and vegetables usually contain 10 to 100 times more salt than fresh or frozen foods, but in recent years many manufacturers have decreased the salt added;
- Fruits canned in heavy syrup contain twice as much sugar as fresh fruits, and the sugar is always refined;
- Some fruits are now available canned in fruit juice, which improves the nutritional content.

Damaged Cans

Damaged or bulging cans are a sign of a chemical change or of bacteria in the can; always discard to avoid poisoning.

If your child's regular diet contains plenty of fresh foods and milk there is no need to avoid all canned foods; handle with care as mentioned above.

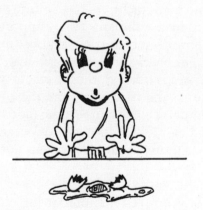

Chapter Twenty-Three

Food Colorings

FOOD COLORINGS ADD COLOR to foods when heat and light have tarnished and discolored them; they standardize the color of foods, eliminating seasonal color variations in butter or in oranges; they improve the general appearance of foods (caramel, for instance, is often used to give a richer, darker color to *brown* breads, cookies, crackers, and gravies); and they give the illusion of the presence of fruit in such products as fruit-flavored drinks, fruit-flavored jellies, fruit-flavored crystals, or lollipops.

Several scientists have attempted to understand the relationship between synthetic food colors and behavioral problems in young children. When Dr. Feingold recommended the elimination of synthetic food colors in his K-P diet, he fueled a whole new debate on this issue.

Some studies have shown that a small percentage of hyperactive children (less than 10 percent) react negatively to synthetic food colors. The behavior of these children tends to improve when these substances are eliminated from their diets. *Tartrazine*, *amaranth*, and *erythrosine* are among the food colors most commonly responsible for allergic reactions.

In Canada the Food and Drug Act allows the use of 24 natural and ten synthetic food colors.

Synthetic Food Colors Currently Permitted in Canada

- allura red (red no 40)
- amaranth (red no 2)
- brilliant blue (blue no 1)
- fast green (green no 3)
- sunset yellow (yellow no 6)
- erythrosine (red no 3)
- tartrazine (yellow no 5)
- indigotine (blue no 2)
- citrus red no 2 (only on orange peels)
- ponceau SX (red no 4, only on candied or glazed fruits and maraschino cherries)

Allergic children who have reacted well to the elimination diet should

1. Limit the consumption of *synthetic food colors* not only in foods, but also in toothpaste and medications, including liquid vitamin supplements and pills. Unfortunately, the hunt for food colors is not always simple: the law on labeling makes it compulsory to mention any food color but not to identify it.

   - The word *natural* before a color means that it comes from a natural source;
   - When the word *color* is used alone, it means that some or all the colors used are synthetic;
   - When in doubt, write to the manufacturer to have the food color identified;
   - If necessary, ask your pharmacist or doctor about the presence of tartrazine in medications that your child takes.

2. Give priority to foods without any added food colors:

   - most cereals and whole grain breads
   - all fresh fruit except orange peel
   - most frozen fruits
   - all fresh vegetables and most frozen vegetables
   - meats, poultry, and fresh or frozen fish
   - legumes and plain tofu
   - fresh, canned, or frozen fruit juices (but always read the label)
   - milk, plain yogurt, and many fruit yogurts
   - nuts and seeds, nut and seed butters except colored pistachios

3. Remember that the more a food is processed, precooked, or sweetened the more likely it is to contain one or more food colors (see chart page 107).

4. Avoid coloring foods at home. The food colors sold in grocery stores in small bottles are all *synthetic*.

The following foods generally contain food colors. Labels mention the presence of food colors but rarely identify them.

cookies, desserts and sweets, and cereal products
commercial chocolate or cream cookies
commercial chocolate or jam cakes
commercial sweetened breakfast cereals (some cereal boxes identify food colors)
instant peach oatmeal
candies and chocolates
chewing gum
candied fruits
maraschino cherries
many jams and jellies
spreads
fruit-flavored gelatine with sugar or aspartame
fruit-flavored crystals for drinks
fruit-flavored drinks
sherbets
pie fillings
cake icings
whipped cream substitutes
topping for sundaes

colored ice cream cups
ready-to-serve puddings
syrups
Popsicles
crackers and chips
pastas with powdered cheese mixes
coating mix for baking

dairy products
cheese spreads
cheese fondue mixes
ice creams
fruit-flavored ice bars

seasonings and other condiments
barbecue sauces
soy sauces
regular relish
mustards
pickles
Chinese cherry sauce
salad dressings
coffee whiteners

Chapter Twenty-Four

Fats

NORTH AMERICANS are digging their own graves by consuming too much fat, but young children should not be on a *low fat diet* too soon in life. Scientific research done in the last 30 years has clearly shown that an excessive intake of fats leads to obesity, cardiovascular diseases, and certain cancers, but researchers are still deliberating the question of when to introduce a child to a lower-fat diet. The impact of the poor quality fats eaten in North America is also under scrutiny. The debate should last well into the 21st century!

A child who learns to eat a moderate amount of fat and who learns to recognize *good* fats from *bad* fats will have healthier eating habits for life.

A child needs the *essential fatty acids* present in foods to develop normally, so there are no grounds for cutting good fats out of his diet; there is, however, a need to balance *quantity* with *quality:*

- Eat whole grain bread without butter or margarine;
- Choose lean fresh meats instead of cold cuts and processed meats;
- Include fish and seafood to get a good supply of omega-3 fatty acids;
- Eat tofu or legumes a few meals a week;
- Offer cheese with less than 20% fat;
- Serve yogurt more often than ice cream;
- Serve partially skimmed milk (2%) after the age of two;
- Limit fried foods;
- Prepare salad dressings from scratch with a good quality cold-pressed oil (olive or sunflower).

A *good* fat is one that provides essential fatty acids in their purest form: sunflower, corn, soya, safflower, canola, and olive oils are good sources, especially when cold-pressed.

A *bad* fat is one that does not provide enough essential fatty acids because of intense heating and/or processing: margarines, fried foods, shortenings, hydrogenated fats, and products that contain such fats.

Foods that are rich in *saturated* fats like butter, meats, and cheeses provide small amounts of essential fatty acids but have been shown to increase the cholesterol levels of high-risk individuals; they cannot be eliminated from a child's diet but should be served in moderation.

Fake fats that provide texture but fewer calories are now found in some ice creams in Canada and in many more foods in the United States; they do not provide essential fatty acids and do not belong in a child's diet.

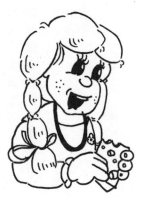

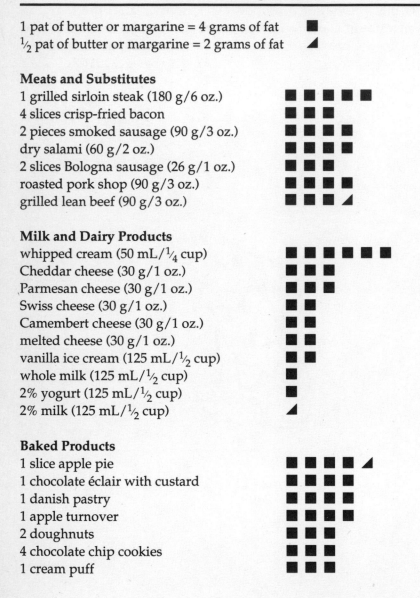

1 pat of butter or margarine = 4 grams of fat

$\frac{1}{2}$ pat of butter or margarine = 2 grams of fat

Meats and Substitutes

1 grilled sirloin steak (180 g/6 oz.)

4 slices crisp-fried bacon

2 pieces smoked sausage (90 g/3 oz.)

dry salami (60 g/2 oz.)

2 slices Bologna sausage (26 g/1 oz.)

roasted pork shop (90 g/3 oz.)

grilled lean beef (90 g/3 oz.)

Milk and Dairy Products

whipped cream (50 mL/$\frac{1}{4}$ cup)

Cheddar cheese (30 g/1 oz.)

Parmesan cheese (30 g/1 oz.)

Swiss cheese (30 g/1 oz.)

Camembert cheese (30 g/1 oz.)

melted cheese (30 g/1 oz.)

vanilla ice cream (125 mL/$\frac{1}{2}$ cup)

whole milk (125 mL/$\frac{1}{2}$ cup)

2% yogurt (125 mL/$\frac{1}{2}$ cup)

2% milk (125 mL/$\frac{1}{2}$ cup)

Baked Products

1 slice apple pie

1 chocolate éclair with custard

1 danish pastry

1 apple turnover

2 doughnuts

4 chocolate chip cookies

1 cream puff

Prepared Foods

1 cup canned chili con carne without beans

1 slice meat pie

1 baked poultry pâté (10 cm/4 in.)

1 egg roll

chicken fried rice (250 mL/1 cup)

1 slice pizza with sausage

Nuts

roasted nuts (125 mL/½ cup)

peanut butter (30 mL/2 tbsp.)

Sweets

20 medium chips

1 chocolate bar

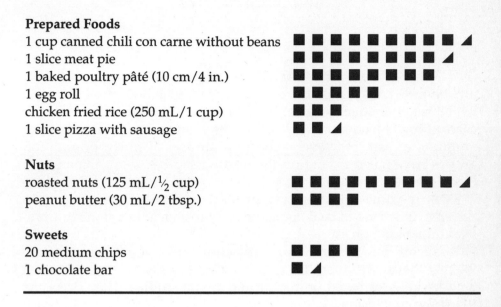

Chapter Twenty-Five

Salt

SALT HAS A BAD REPUTATION because it contains a lot of *sodium* and because research has linked sodium to high blood pressure.

For years, epidemiologists have been saying that there are more cases of high blood pressure in countries where people consume large amounts of salt. However, thorough studies of given population groups have failed to confirm the relationship between salt and high blood pressure.

Even if a low-salt diet may prove beneficial in treating some patients, it has yet to be demonstrated that such a diet alone can prevent high blood pressure.

While the media is running antisodium campaigns, scientists are looking for causes other than salt. In recent years, they have proposed new hypotheses based on recent nutritional studies. They drew the following conclusions:

- An increased intake of potassium (fruit and vegetables) lowers the chances of developing high blood pressure;
- Other nutrients such as calcium and vitamins A and C also lower chances of high blood pressure;
- The link with sodium has never been confirmed.

These new findings imply new additions to the diet rather than the simple subtraction of salt. They suggest a diet with more fruits, vegetables, and milk at any age (see Appendix A for sources of potassium, calcium, and sodium).

These new findings should be considered guidelines, not definitive answers.

However, there are advantages to a moderate salt intake: you can learn to enjoy the true flavors of foods. A moderate consumption of salt means

- Seasoning with herbs, garlic, or onions instead of tons of salt;
- Serving fresh foods more often than canned vegetables, meats, or poultry;
- Giving priority to foods that are the least processed.

Chapter Twenty-Six

Sugar

THE AVERAGE CANADIAN eats more than 40 kilos (88 lbs.) of sugar a year, honey and maple products included, which makes a daily average of about 135 mL (9 tbsp.) or 400 vitamin-free calories!

This is much too much!

These figures do not even take into account high fructose corn syrup, the new sweetener made from corn syrup and used extensively by the food industry to sweeten drinks and canned products, but not declared in consumer statistics.

What happens to the young child living in this world of sugar addicts? Can he afford to imitate his parents and remain healthy?

A child does not need candy, cakes, jams, cookies, or sweetened drinks to grow and have energy. Her body can easily process fruit, milk, bread, and vegetables into glucose, which becomes the sugar-fuel needed to function properly. In fact, her body works more efficiently with less refined sugar.

- A child who eats a lot of sweet foods is not as hungry for vitamin- and fiber-rich foods. He may even develop an iron deficiency or lack dietary fiber; anemia, constipation, and even hypoglycemia are possible side effects;
- A child who snacks on cookies and sweets between meals, who drinks fruit juices all day long, is clearing the way for dental caries and will spend many painful hours in the dentist's chair;
- A child for whom desserts, cakes, or chocolates are the supreme reward may end up giving sugar too much importance and slowly become sugar-dependent;
- A two-year-old who learns to enjoy most foods with little or no added sugar is not really deprived of sugar. You only miss what you know well!
- A five- or six-year-old used to finding sugar in everything he eats, can hardly appreciate a plain grapefruit, yogurt with fresh fruits, strawberries without sugar, toast without jam, plain milk without chocolate.

Sugar does not need to become a forbidden food, but it should be given less importance in our diets and those of our children.

Everybody knows that soft drinks and fruit-flavored drinks and jellies are highly sweetened foods, but do you have any idea how much sugar these foods dump into your body per year?

Here are the facts!

- A can of cola per day provides 13 kg (28 lb.) of sugar per year!
- A large glass of a colored and sweetened fruit-flavored drink provides 14 kg (30 lb.) of sugar per year!
- A large bowl of fruit-flavored jelly per day provides 15 kilos (34 lb.) of sugar per year!

When giving up sugar, pay extra attention to *hidden* sugars because 75 percent of all the sugar you actually eat is hidden in processed foods (see chart on page 115).

Remember that the younger your child is, the easier it is to learn the following good habits:

- Live with less *added* sugar;
- Drink water or diluted fruit juices instead of sweetened drinks and colas;
- Snack on fruit or cheese instead of candy;
- Enjoy unsweetened cereal instead of cereal-flavored candies;
- Crunch into some raw veggies, a cracker, a piece of toasted bread instead of a sweet or chocolate-flavored cookie;
- Use peanut butter, applesauce, banana slices, or fruit purée instead of jams or marmalade on bread;
- Choose yogurt or fruit-juice jellies instead of sweetened puddings or fruit-flavored jellies.

Getting your child accustomed to less sugar means

- Helping him discover the whole range of flavors in gorgeous vegetables, ripe fruits, and whole grains;
- Preventing long-term sugar dependency and all the problems associated with it.

But it does not mean that your child cannot enjoy the occasional sweet!

1 tsp. sugar = 4g   4 g = ▉   2 g = ▪   1 g = ▪

Hidden sugar
Milk and Dairy Products
chocolate milk
  250 mL (1 cup)
fruit yogurt
  100 g (3½ oz.)

Vegetables
cream-style corn
  250 mL (1 cup)
canned peas
  250 mL (1 cup)

Fruits and Fruit Juices
frozen strawberries with sugar
  125 mL (½ cup)
frozen raspberries with sugar
  125 mL (½ cup)
applesauce, sweetened,
  125 mL (½ cup)
pineapple, canned with syrup
  125 mL (½ cup)
apricots, canned, with syrup,
  125 mL (½ cup)
peaches, canned, with syrup,
  125 mL (½ cup)
pears, canned, with syrup,
  125 mL (½ cup)
fruit salad, canned, with syrup
  125 mL (½ cup)
prunes, canned, with syrup
  125 mL (½ cup)
cherries, canned, with syrup
  125 mL (½ cup)
grapefruit juice, sweetened
  250 mL (1 cup)

maraschino cherries, 6 large
    (50g/2 oz.)

cranberries, in sauce
    15 mL (1 tbsp)

orange juice, sweetened
    250 mL (1 cup)

Breakfast Cereal

Sugar Corn Pops
    28 g (¾ cup)

Frosted Flakes
    28 g (1 cup)

Honey Nuts
    28 g (¾ cup)

instant oatmeal, maple flavor
    250 mL (1 cup) cooked

Bran and Raisin Bites
    28 g (½ cup)

Raisin Bran
    28 g (½ cup)

Bran Flakes with fruit
    28 g (⅔ cup)

Shreddies
    28 g (⅝ cup)

Kellogg's Pep
    28 g (⅔ cup)

Bran Flakes
    28 g (⅔ cup)

Special K
    28 g (1 cup)

Rice Krispies
    28 g (1 cup)

Corn Flakes
    28 g (1 cup)

Drinks

orange, cherry, grape drinks
 250 mL (1 cup)
cream soda
 250 mL (1 cup)
root beer
 250 mL (1 cup)
cola
 250 mL (1 cup)
ginger ale
 250 mL (1 cup)
lemonade, sweetened
 250 mL (1 cup)
instant chocolate drink powder
 1 tbsp (30 mL)

Others

1 Popsicle
Jell-O
 125 mL (½ cup)
caramel popcorn
 125 mL (½ cup)
chewing gum with sugar, 1 piece

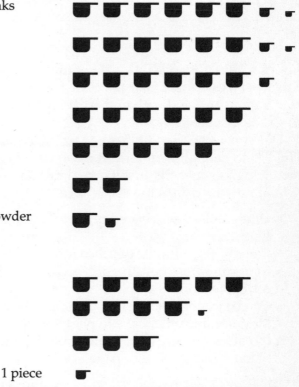

Chapter Twenty-Seven

Fruit Juices and Fruit-Flavored Drinks

OUR CHILDREN DRINK a lot of juice — approximately 36 L (9 gallons) per year. Too much juice! In fact, Canadians in general drink much more juice today than they did ten years ago. It is not necessary to drink so much juice.

Did you know that a 125 mL (4 oz.) glass of orange juice provides a child with enough vitamin C for two days? One or two glasses a day are enough to quench thirst. Beyond this amount, the advantages fade.

A child who drinks too much juice

- Often refuses to drink enough milk, a much more important food;
- Can develop chronic diarrhea (see Chapter 13);
- Can suffer from constipation because by drinking instead of eating her fruits she misses out on dietary fiber;
- Can be hungry more often because liquids are not filling;
- May, if vulnerable, have hypoglycemic reactions because juice is transformed very quickly into sugar, which temporarily raises blood sugar levels (see page 71).

To wean a child who loves juice any hour of the day

- Gradually dilute juice by adding a little more water every day until the proportion is 50/50;
- Serve water instead of juice at meals and give milk at the end of meals; offer diluted juice only after fruit or a solid snack.

Chapter Twenty-Eight

Chocolate

CHOCOLATE HOLDS A SPECIAL PLACE in the hearts of many people young and old, and I have no intention of challenging this special bond. I just want to provide some data on the composition of chocolate and its rival, *carob*.

Classic chocolate is made with cocoa paste, cocoa butter, and sugar, and it may contain milk, nuts, fruits, and flavorings, depending on the product.

Chocolate contains several nutrients: some protein, saturated fat, minerals, and theobromine, a stimulant similar to caffeine.

Chocolate is a treat and does not belong in the child's regular diet because of its high fat content, refined sugar, and stimulant. And it can cause allergic reactions in some children. Because of these problems, you should use other delicious products instead.

For many years, *carob* has been used as a chocolate substitute. It is derived from the dry pod of the carob tree, which grows in hot climates. Available in health food stores, carob contains nutrients, more carbohydrates, and less fat than cocoa; it is not allergenic and contains no stimulants.

Carob has a very pleasant flavor but does not taste like cocoa even though its color is similar. If you want to use carob instead of chocolate in a recipe you will have to experiment. As a general rule

$$\underset{\text{45 mL (3 tbsp.)}}{\text{carob}} + \underset{\text{30 mL (2 tbsp.)}}{\text{liquid}} = \underset{\text{1 square 30 g (1 oz.)}}{\text{unsweetened chocolate}}$$

The few advantages of carob over chocolate do not mean that it can be used every day. Carob should also remain a treat.

PART 4

Tamed Recipes

"*I still think that one of the pleasantest of all emotions is to know that I, I with my brain and my hands, have nourished my beloved few, that I have concocted a stew or a story, a rarity or a plain dish, to sustain them truly against the hungers of the world.*"

M. F. K. FISHER

The Gastronomical Me

Nutritional Values of Recipes

★ ★ ★   6–9 mg of iron per serving

★ ★   3–5 mg of iron per serving

★   1–2 mg of iron per serving

90 g (3 oz.) of meat, fish, or poultry

60 g (2oz.) of meat, fish, or poultry

30 g (1oz.) of meat, fish, or poultry

15 g (½ oz) of meat, fish, or poultry

50–75 mg of vitamin C per serving

30–49 mg of vitamin C per serving

300 and over ER of vitamin A per serving

170–299 ER of vitamin A per serving

120–169 ER of vitamin A per serving

2–4 mg of dietary fiber per serving

275–330 mg of calcium per serving

197–274 mg of calcium per serving

119–196 mg of calcium per serving

40–118 mg of calcium per serving

For example, a recipe with the following symbols

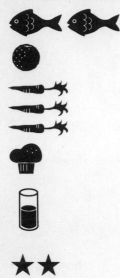 contains as much protein as 60 g or 2 oz. of meat

contains as much vitamin C as one small orange

contains as much vitamin A as 3 small carrots

contains as much fiber as 1 bran muffin

contains as much calcium as 125 mL (4 oz.) glass of milk

 contains 3 to 4 mg of iron

Key to Recipe Classification

 recipe without meat

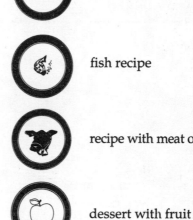 breakfast recipe

 recipe without sugar

fish recipe

 recipe without corn

recipe with meat or chicken

 recipe without eggs

dessert with fruit

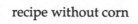 recipe without wheat

 recipe without milk or dairy products

 recipe without chocolate

 recipe for BBQ

 recipe with vegetables

Breakfast Treats

Peanut Butter Squares

1 egg
1 large banana
125 mL ($\frac{1}{2}$ cup) peanut butter
45 mL (3 tbsp.) raisins
250 mL (1 cup) oatmeal
125 mL ($\frac{1}{2}$ cup) coconut, unsweetened
75 mL ($\frac{1}{3}$ cup) unhulled sesame seeds

Cream first 4 ingredients in blender or with mixer. Pour into a bowl and mix in remaining ingredients.

Pour mixture into a greased square cake pan, 20 x 20 cm (8 x 8 in.). Bake about 25 minutes in 180°C (350°F) oven, until edges pull away from sides of pan. Makes 16 squares.

1 square provides

protein

Buckwheat Pancakes

375 mL (1½ cups) buckwheat flour
125 mL (½ cup) oat bran
2 mL (½ tsp.) salt
2 mL (½ tsp.) baking powder
500 mL (2 cups) apple juice
45 mL (3 tbsp.) maple syrup or honey
15 mL (1 tbsp.) soy or sunflower oil

In a bowl, mix together all dry ingredients. In separate bowl, combine liquid ingredients and add to dry ones. Stir well.

Cook on a greased skillet using 45 mL (3 tbsp.) batter for each pancake. Makes 10 to 12 pancakes.

Each pancake provides

iron

Granola Special

250 mL (1 cup) oatmeal
45 mL (3 tbsp.) oat bran
45 mL (3 tbsp.) sunflower seeds
75 mL (5 tbsp.) raisins
75 mL (5 tbsp.) chopped dates
75 mL (5 tbsp.) chopped almonds
15 mL (1 tbsp.) honey or maple syrup
15 mL (1 tbsp.) sunflower oil

Preheat oven to 200°C (400°F).

Spread oatmeal and oat bran on a cookie sheet and toast until golden. Stir every minute for about 5 minutes. Add sunflower seeds, raisins, dates, and almonds. Toast for another 5 minutes. Add honey and oil, stir and toast 5 more minutes.

Remove from oven. When cooled store in a loosely closed jar. Makes 500 mL (2 cups).

Each portion with 125 mL (¹⁄₂ cup) milk added provides

   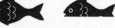

iron   **protein**

Mini Fruit Pancakes

500 mL (2 cups) whole wheat flour
250 mL (1 cup) iron-fortified infant cereal
15 mL (1 tbsp.) baking powder
15 mL (1 tbsp.) brown sugar
5 mL (1 tsp.) salt
2 mL ($\frac{1}{2}$ tsp.) cinnamon
625 mL ($2\frac{1}{2}$ cups) partially skimmed milk
1 egg
45 mL (3 tbsp.) oil
juice of half a lemon
125 mL ($\frac{1}{2}$ cup) fresh or frozen fruits, unsweetened (peaches, strawberries, blueberries)

On a large sheet of waxed paper, combine all dry ingredients, except fruits. In a large bowl, mix milk, egg, oil, and lemon juice. Add solid ingredients to liquid ingredients and stir lightly; carefully fold in fruits.

Cook on a preheated and greased skillet for 3 to 4 minutes. Makes about 20 small pancakes.

Each pancake provides

protein   iron

Date Bread

375 mL (1½ cups) whole wheat cake flour
5 mL (1 tsp.) baking powder
5 mL (1 tsp.) salt
5 mL (1 tsp.) baking soda
175 mL (⅔ cup) boiling apple juice
250 mL (1 cup) chopped dates
45 mL (3 tbsp.) butter
75 mL (5 tbsp.) maple syrup or honey
1 egg
5 mL (1 tsp.) vanilla
125 mL (½ cup) chopped nuts

In a bowl, combine flour, baking powder, and salt. In another bowl, dissolve baking soda in boiling apple juice and pour over dates.

With mixer, blend butter and syrup (honey) until creamy. Add egg and vanilla. Add dry ingredients to this mixture alternately with cooled dates and juice. Add chopped nuts.

Pour mixture into loaf pan. Bake 45 to 55 minutes in 180°C (350°F) oven. Makes 22, 1 cm (½ in.) slices.

Each portion provides

iron

Apple Pancakes

375 mL (1½ cups) 2% milk
250 mL (1 cup) oatmeal
30 mL (2 tbsp.) oil
2 eggs, beaten
15 mL (1 tbsp.) honey or maple syrup
250 mL (1 cup) whole wheat flour
5 mL (1 tsp.) baking powder
1 mL (¼ tsp.) salt
dash ground nutmeg
1 apple, grated

In a bowl, combine oatmeal and milk, and let stand for 5 minutes. Add oil, eggs, and honey, and stir well.

In another bowl, combine flour, baking powder, salt, and spices. Add to liquids. Stir in grated apple.

Cook on a lightly greased skillet using 45 mL (3 tbsp.) of batter for each pancake. Makes 14 pancakes.

Each pancake provides

protein   fiber   iron

Irresistible Vegetable Dishes

Carrots *en Papillotte* on the BBQ

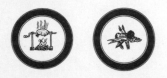

3 or 4 carrots, cut into narrow strips
15 mL (1 tbsp.) chopped parsley
15 mL (1 tbsp.) butter
5 mL (1 tsp.) lemon juice
salt and pepper to taste
2 large, thick sheets of aluminum foil, stacked

Place carrot sticks on foil, add parsley, butter, lemon juice, salt, and pepper.

Wrap loosely, and seal with double folds. Cook 8 cm (3 in.) over a coal fire 30 to 45 minutes, or until carrots are tender. Turn the package over once. Makes 6 to 8 portions.

Each portion provides

vitamin A

Corn-on-the-Cob *en Papillotte*

1 ear of corn
1 piece of thick aluminum foil
butter
salt and pepper to taste

Peel back outer husks almost to the base and remove silk. Place ear on foil and brush with butter. Sprinkle with salt and pepper.

Wrap husk back over corn. Wrap corn in foil and seal tightly, twisting ends. Grill 25 to 30 minutes, turning often.

Each portion provides

fiber

Vegetables in a Glass

500 mL (2 cups) tomato juice
250 mL (1 cup) alfalfa sprouts
juice of 1 lime or ½ lemon

Mix juice and alfalfa sprouts in a blender until sprouts are liquified. Add lemon juice. Pour into chilled glasses and serve immediately. Makes 3 to 4 portions.

Each portion provides

vitamin C

Grapefruit-Zucchini Drink

500 mL (2 cups) grapefruit juice
2 small zucchini
rosemary, to taste

Wash zucchini well but don't peel. Cut off ends and slice.

Purée with other ingredients in blender until smooth. Check seasoning and add rosemary if desired.

Pour into chilled glasses and serve immediately. Makes 4 portions.

Each portion provides

vitamin C

Basil Delight

250 mL (1 cup) tomato juice
8 fresh basil leaves
juice of half a lemon

Purée all ingredients in blender until smooth. Add 1 or 2 ice cubes and blend until foamy. Serve chilled. Makes 2 to 3 portions.

Each portion provides

vitamin C

Parsley Surprise

500 mL (2 cups) pineapple juice
375 mL (1½ cups) fresh parsley

Mix in blender until homogeneous. Pour into chilled glasses and serve immediately. Makes 4 to 6 portions.

Each portion provides

vitamin C

Cheesy Potato

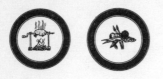

1 potato
30 mL (2 tbsp.) shredded cheese
5 mL (1 tsp.) parsley
5 mL (1 tsp.) butter
salt and pepper
1 sheet of aluminum foil

Wash and scrub potato. Cut into halves. Remove a big spoonful of flesh from each half. Stuff each half with cheese, parsley, butter, salt and pepper. Wrap both halves in foil. Bake 1 hour. Turn over often.

Each portion provides

fiber

Apple-Turnip Soup

5 mL (1 tsp.) oil
1 chopped onion
1 small turnip, diced
2 apples, peeled and diced
500 mL (2 cups) chicken broth
2 mL ($\frac{1}{2}$ tsp.) salt
1 mL ($\frac{1}{4}$ tsp.) pepper
1 mL ($\frac{1}{4}$ tsp.) nutmeg
500 mL (2 cups) milk (use water for a recipe without milk)
125 mL ($\frac{1}{2}$ cup) chopped parsley

In a large saucepan, heat oil and add onion, cooking until soft. Add turnip, apples, broth, salt, pepper, and nutmeg.

Cover and simmer about 35 minutes or until turnip is tender. Allow to cool, then purée in blender.

Season to taste. Before serving, stir in milk and warm the soup. Garnish with parsley. Makes 8 portions.

Each portion provides

calcium

Pumpkin Soup

1 kg (2 lb.) pumpkin, cut into big chunks
1 onion, cut into 8 pieces
750 mL (3 cups) chicken broth
30 mL (2 tbsp.) ginger, freshly grated
or 2 mL (½ tsp.) ground dried ginger
1 mL (¼ tsp.) cinnamon
salt and pepper, freshly ground
250 mL (1 cup) plain yogurt

Put all ingredients except yogurt into a large saucepan, and bring to a boil. Reduce heat and simmer 15 minutes or until pumpkin is tender.

Remove from heat and purée in blender. Return mixture to saucepan, reheat. Add yogurt just before serving.

For special occasions, use a cleaned out pumpkin for a tureen or serve in small winter squashes. Makes about 8 small portions.

Each portion provides

vitamin A

Carrot Soup

30 mL (2 tbsp.) butter
750 mL (3 cups) carrots, chopped
500 mL (2 cups) water or vegetable cooking water
2 mL ($\frac{1}{2}$ tsp.) ginger
30 mL (2 tbsp.) parsley, chopped
250 mL (1 cup) 2% milk (optional)
15 mL (1 tbsp.) green onions, finely chopped

Sauté carrots in butter until lightly browned. Add water and herbs and cover. Simmer until carrots are tender.

Purée carrots in blender. Reheat and add milk and green onions. Makes 16 portions of 125 mL ($\frac{1}{2}$ cup).

Each portion provides

vitamin A

Coleslaw, Apple, and Cheese

$\frac{1}{4}$ small green cabbage, shredded
75 mL (5 tbsp.) celery, chopped
30 mL (2 tbsp.) green onions, finely chopped
30 mL (2 tbsp.) mayonnaise
30 mL (2 tbsp.) yogurt
7 mL ($1\frac{1}{2}$ tsp.) lemon juice
salt and pepper to taste
dash fennel seeds
1 medium apple, diced
45 mL (3 tbsp.) cheddar cheese, diced

In a bowl, combine cabbage, celery, and green onions. In a small bowl, mix mayonnaise, yogurt, lemon juice, salt, pepper, and fennel seeds. Add to cabbage mixture and toss. Refrigerate 2 to 3 hours.

Before serving add diced apple and cheddar cheese, mix well. Makes 4 portions.

Each portion provides

calcium

Mouth-Watering Main Dishes

Tuna-Cheeseburger

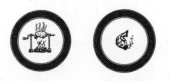

1 whole wheat English muffin, halved
1 egg
90 g (3 oz.) tuna
15 mL (1 tbsp.) plain yogurt
30 mL (2 tbsp.) cheddar or mozzarella cheese, shredded
salt and pepper to taste
1 sheet of aluminum foil

In a bowl, combine egg, tuna, and yogurt. Add salt and pepper to taste. Spread mixture on each half of English muffin. Sprinkle with cheddar cheese. Wrap in foil and prick with a fork. Grill 5 minutes. Makes 2 portions.

Each portion provides

protein

Barbecued Fish Kabob

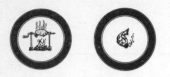

125 g (¼ lb.) scallops
250 g (½ lb.) raw shrimp, shelled
125 g (¼ lb.) turbot or sole, cut into 6 chunks
6 mushroom caps
1 onion, cut into large chunks

Marinade
30 mL (2 tbsp.) vegetable oil
60 mL (4 tbsp.) lemon juice
1 onion, minced
15 mL (1 tbsp.) parsley, chopped
5 mL (1 tsp.) thyme
1 bay leaf
dash of pepper
2 garlic cloves, minced

Prepare marinade in small bowl. Add kabob ingredients and marinate one hour in the refrigerator, stirring occasionally.

On 6 skewers, thread scallops alternately with onions, shrimp, mushrooms, and turbot.

Grill about 13 cm (5 in.) over coals for about 10 minutes, turning and basting with marinade frequently. Makes 6 kabobs.

Each portion provides

protein

Salmon Croquettes

45 mL (3 tbsp.) onion, minced
3 green onions, thinly sliced
10 mL (2 tsp.) butter
190 g (6 ½ oz.) fresh or canned salmon
250 mL (1 cup) cottage cheese
1 egg
250 mL (1 cup) whole wheat bread crumbs
5 mL (1 tsp.) dried thyme
salt and pepper to taste
béchamel or tartar sauce

In a small pan, sauté onion and green onions in butter until soft.

In a large bowl or food processor mix all other ingredients; add onions and check seasoning.

Place about 45 mL (3 tbsp.) on a greased cookie sheet and bake about 20 minutes in a 180°C (350°F) oven. Serve with béchamel or homemade tartar sauce. Makes 16 to 18 small croquettes.

Each croquette provides

protein

Wild Zucchini

4 small zucchini
250 mL (1 cup) chick peas, cooked
1 small onion, thinly sliced
1 clove garlic
5 mL (1 tsp.) corn oil
5 mL (1 tsp.) dry thyme
250 mL (1 cup) mozzarella cheese, shredded
45 mL (3 tbsp.) wheat germ

Wash zucchini and halve lengthwise; scoop out flesh and reserve for stuffing. Place zucchini shells on a small cookie sheet.

Chop zucchini flesh. Mash chick peas and combine with zucchini. Sauté garlic and onion in the oil until soft. Add to zucchini and chick peas. Add thyme and check seasoning.

Stuff zucchini, cover with foil, and bake about 30 minutes in a 180°C (350°F) oven, or until zucchini are tender. Remove from oven, sprinkle with shredded cheese and wheat germ, and return to oven. Grill until cheese is melted. Makes 8 portions.

Each portion provides

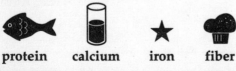

protein   calcium   iron   fiber

Fettuccine with Tuna and Vegetables

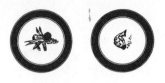

250 mL (1 cup) zucchini
250 mL (1 cup) broccoli, cut into small florets
1 190 g (6½ oz.) can tuna
625 mL (2½ cups) spinach fettuccine, cooked "al dente"

Cheese Sauce
30 mL (2 tbsp.) butter
30 mL (2 tbsp.) whole wheat flour
1 mL (¼ tsp.) mustard powder
250 mL (1 cup) 2% milk
250 mL (1 cup) mozzarella, shredded
125 mL (½ cup) cheddar, shredded
salt and pepper

Steam vegetables for about 5 minutes.

Meanwhile prepare sauce. Melt butter in a saucepan. Combine flour and mustard powder and add to melted butter. Gradually stir in milk and cook over medium heat until mixture thickens, stirring constantly. Remove from heat and add shredded cheese, salt, and pepper. Makes about 180 mL (1¾ cups) cheese sauce.

Add vegetables and tuna to cheese sauce. Mix well and reheat. Add hot pasta and serve. Makes 8 portions.

Each portion provides

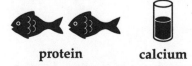

protein   calcium

Fettuccine Florentine

300 g (10 oz.) fresh spinach
45 mL (3 tbsp.) onion, grated
15 mL (1 tbsp.) butter
125 mL (½ cup) milk
1 egg, lightly beaten
250 mL (1 cup) feta cheese, crumbled
250 mL (1 cup) cottage cheese
nutmeg and pepper to taste
240 g (8 oz.) uncooked or 1 L (4 cups) cooked spinach or egg noodles

Wash and drain spinach and place into saucepan. Cover and cook over high heat until the lid becomes hot, then lower heat and cook 3 to 5 minutes until wilted. Strain and chop finely.

In a large skillet, sauté onion in butter until transparent. Add spinach and cook for a few minutes. Remove from heat and allow to cool a little. Add egg, milk, cheeses, and seasoning. Mix well and heat to warm. Pour over hot noodles, toss, and serve. Makes 8 portions.

Each portion provides

protein

★
iron

calcium

Cheese Fondue

375 mL (1½ cups) raw vegetables, diced (broccoli and cauliflower florets, carrots, mushrooms, green and red peppers, zucchini)
125 mL (½ cup) cottage cheese
125 mL (½ cup) 2% milk
15 mL (1 tbsp.) butter
½ garlic clove (optional)
2 mL (½ tsp.) mustard powder
1 mL (¼ tsp.) nutmeg
15 mL (1 tbsp.) corn starch
200 mL (¾ cup) Swiss cheese, shredded
whole wheat bread chunks

Steam vegetables about 5 minutes (except for mushrooms, peppers, zucchini).

Blend cottage cheese and 45 mL (3 tbsp.) milk in blender.

In a saucepan, melt butter, add garlic, mustard, and nutmeg. Cook about 1 minute over medium heat. Stir in starch, cottage cheese, and rest of milk and cook until it thickens. Lower heat and stir in Swiss cheese until it melts.

Pour into a fondue pot. Serve with bread and vegetables. Makes 6 portions.

Each portion provides

protein   **calcium**

Grilled Cheese Sandwich

2 slices whole wheat bread
1 slice cheese
butter (optional)
tomato slices (optional)

Lightly butter each slice of whole wheat bread. Place cheese on unbuttered side of one slice. Place other slice on top.

Barbecue or toast under grill in oven until golden, turn, and repeat.

Some tomato slices may be added at the end, if desired. Makes 2 portions.

Each portion provides

protein

Shrimp Paella

30 mL (2 tbsp.) olive oil
½ onion, thinly sliced
1 garlic clove, minced
½ green pepper
125 mL (½ cup) brown rice, soaked 30 minutes in cold water and
    strained
175 mL (⅔ cup) vegetable broth
1 large tomato, blanched, peeled, seeded, and chopped
125 mL (½ cup) frozen peas
dash saffron
½ small chicken, cut into 4 pieces
120 g (4 oz.) shrimp

Sauté chicken in oil until nicely browned, remove, and put on a plate. Add onion, garlic, and pepper to pan and sauté 5 to 7 minutes. Add rice and cook 5 minutes, stirring frequently. Pour in broth, bring to a boil, then reduce heat. Add rest of ingredients and chicken.

Bake about 30 minutes in a 180°C (350°F) oven or until rice is done. Makes 4 to 5 portions.

Each portion provides

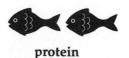

   protein

Stuffed Pita Bread

1 whole wheat pita bread
125 mL (½ cup) chicken, cooked and diced
45 mL (3 tbsp.) mozzarella cheese, diced
1 tomato, diced
45 mL (3 tbsp.) mushrooms, sliced
alfalfa or lettuce
30 mL (2 tbsp.) yogurt salad dressing (recipe below)

Open one end of pita and stuff with chicken, cheese, tomato, and mushrooms.

Grill until golden. Add alfalfa or lettuce and salad dressing. Cut in half. Makes 2 portions.

Yogurt Dressing
5 mL (1 tsp.) Dijon mustard
15 mL (1 tbsp.) cider vinegar
10 mL (2 tsp.) honey
175 mL (⅔ cup) plain yogurt
50 mL (3 tbsp.) mayonnaise
salt and pepper to taste

Mix ingredients and store, covered, in refrigerator. Makes 250 mL (1 cup).

Each portion provides

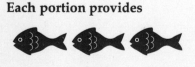

protein

Meat Loaf in Disguise

250 g (½ lb.) lean ground beef
45 mL (3 tbsp.) oatmeal
60 mL (4 tbsp.) wheat germ
125 mL (½ cup) chick peas
30 mL (2 tbsp.) onion, minced
¼ of 156 mL (5½ oz.) can tomato paste
1 egg
salt and pepper to taste

Mash chick peas with fork and combine with all other ingredients. Press into loaf pan.

Bake about 1 hour in a 180°C (350°F) oven. Makes 5 portions. Serve with Fresh Tomato Coulis (see next recipe).

Each portion provides

★★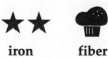

iron   fiber

Fresh Tomato Coulis

1 clove garlic, minced
45 mL (3 tbsp.) onion, minced
15 mL (1 tbsp.) olive oil
2 or 3 ripe tomatoes
5 mL (1 tsp.) dried thyme
salt and pepper to taste
vegetable cooking water or chicken broth (optional)

Sauté garlic and onion in oil until soft. Dice tomatoes and add garlic, onion and thyme.

Cook over low heat for about 10 minutes or until mixture thickens. Remove from heat and blend until smooth in the blender. Check seasoning and add salt and pepper. If sauce is too thick, add 30 mL (2 tbsp.) or 15 mL (1 tbsp.) vegetable cooking water. Makes 250 mL (1 cup).

Shepherd's Pie with Added Vitamins

250 g (¹⁄₂ lb.) lean ground beef
250 mL (1 cup) red lentils, uncooked
3 carrots, finely sliced
375 mL (1¹⁄₂ cups) chicken broth
1 large onion, finely chopped
1 large pepper, finely chopped
10 mL (2 tsp.) oil
30 mL (2 tbsp.) fresh parsley, chopped
392 g (14 oz.) can cream style corn
salt and pepper to taste
4 large potatoes, peeled and quartered
milk and butter to taste

In a medium saucepan, pour broth. Add lentils and carrots and cook 10 to 15 minutes, or until liquid is almost absorbed and lentils and carrots are tender.

In another saucepan, steam potatoes 10 to 20 minutes, until very tender. Remove from heat and mash with a little milk and butter.

While potatoes are cooling, sauté onion and pepper in oil until soft. Add ground beef and cook until meat is brown. Add parsley and season to taste.

Combine cooked lentils with beef-vegetable mixture. Add creamed corn and pour into a baking pan. Cover with mashed potatoes. Bake about 45 minutes in a 180°C (350°F) oven. Serve hot with a little coleslaw or green salad. Makes 8 to 10 portions.

Each portion provides

protein   iron

Fortified Little Pâtés

300 g (10 oz.) pork liver
500 g (1 lb.) lean ground beef
1 egg
1 small potato, grated
125 mL ($\frac{1}{2}$ cup) fortified cream of wheat, uncooked
1 onion, minced
5 mL (1 tsp.) salt
pepper, freshly ground
15 mL (1 tbsp.) Dijon mustard
30 mL (2 tbsp.) tomato paste

Chop the raw pork liver in a blender or food processor. In a large bowl, combine the rest of the ingredients and add the chopped pork. Pour mixture into small, greased muffin pans. Pâtés can be frozen at this stage.

To serve, bake 40 to 60 minutes in a 180°C (350°F) oven. If pâtés have not been frozen, reduce baking time to about 30 minutes. Serve with Fresh Tomato Coulis (see recipe index) or a homemade marinade. Makes 12 small pâtés.

Each little pâté provides

★★★

   iron

Minute Pizza

300 mL (1¼ cups) whole wheat cake flour
dash of salt
45 mL (3 tbsp.) oil
45 mL (3 tbsp.) water
125 mL (½ cup) tomato sauce
120 g (4 oz.) mozzarella cheese, shredded
300 mL (1¼ cups) vegetables, finely sliced (peppers, mushrooms, zucchini, broccoli, celery, etc.)
30 mL (2 tbsp.) Parmesan cheese, grated

In a medium bowl, combine flour and salt. In a measuring cup, combine oil and water. Make a well in the center of the dry ingredients and pour in liquid mixture. Stir with a fork and work into a round ball.

Spread dough with fingers on a 23-cm (9-in.) pie plate or roll with a rolling pin. Dough should not extend more than 2.5 cm (1 in.) up the sides. Bake 15 minutes in a 190°C (375°F) oven and remove.

Top with tomato sauce, vegetables and shredded cheese. Finish with Parmesan.

Bake 10 to 15 minutes in a 190°C (375°F) oven. Makes about 6 portions.

Each portion provides

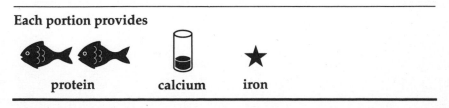

protein   calcium   iron

Lentil and Apple Soup

1 large onion, minced
1 large apple, peeled and thinly sliced
15 mL (1 tbsp.) butter
15 mL (1 tbsp.) oil
30 mL (2 tbsp.) flour
1 L (4 cups) chicken broth or vegetable cooking water
250 mL (1 cup) red lentils, uncooked
30 mL (2 tbsp.) parsley, finely chopped
salt and pepper

Sauté onion and apple in butter and oil for a few minutes, then stir in flour. Add chicken broth gradually and bring to a boil. Add lentils and simmer 30 minutes. Sprinkle with parsley and season with salt and pepper to taste. Makes 8 small portions.

Each portion provides

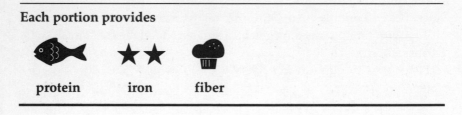

protein   iron   fiber

Chicken with Almonds

30 mL (2 tbsp.) oil
500 mL (2 cups) chicken, cooked
250 mL (1 cup) carrots, thinly sliced
250 mL (1 cup) broccoli florets or green beans, cut into 2.5 cm (1 in.)
   pieces
250 mL (1 cup) cauliflower florets
125 mL (½ cup) green onions, chopped
10 mL (2 tsp.) corn starch
1 clove garlic
125 mL (½ cup) almonds, chopped
250 mL (1 cup) chicken broth

Cook carrots and beans or broccoli in oil for 2 minutes. Add cauli-flower and green onions and cook for another minute. Add chicken broth, corn starch, and garlic and cook until mixture thickens.

Add chicken and almonds, stirring to warm. Makes 8 portions.

Each portion provides

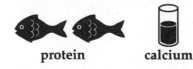

protein   calcium

Mystery Quenelles with Veal Liver

1½ slices whole wheat bread
60 mL (4 tbsp.) milk
125 mL (½ cup) onion, thinly sliced
1 clove garlic, minced
10 mL (2 tsp.) oil
180 g (6 oz.) calf's liver
2 slices bacon, cut into small pieces
30 mL (2 tbsp.) parsley, finely chopped
salt and pepper
45 mL (3 tbsp.) whole wheat flour
1 egg
dash of nutmeg

In a blender or food processor, chop bread into crumbs, put into a small bowl, and add milk.

In a skillet, brown garlic and onion in oil, over low heat, 3 to 4 minutes only. Pour mixture into blender bowl; add liver, bacon, parsley, salt, and pepper. Purée; add flour, egg, nutmeg, and soaked bread; blend a few seconds.

Pour into a large saucepan 5 cm (2 in.) water; simmer but do not boil. Place 50 mL (¼ cup) mixture into simmering water for each quenelle. Poach 10 to 12 minutes. Remove with a slotted spoon and allow to drain well. Cover and keep warm in 150°C (300°F) oven. Serve with Fresh Tomato Coulis (see recipe index). Makes 10 quenelles.

Quenelles can be refrigerated for 2 to 3 days. Warm in oven before serving.

Each quenelle provides

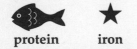

protein   iron

Spinach Quiche

Crust
200 mL (³⁄₄ cup) whole wheat flour
45 mL (3 tbsp.) wheat germ
dash of salt
45 mL (3 tbsp.) oil
30 mL (2 tbsp.) cold water

Filling
2 eggs
240 g (8 oz.) tofu
300 g (10 oz.) package fresh spinach
2 mL ($\frac{1}{2}$ tsp.) nutmeg
125 mL ($\frac{1}{2}$ cup) onion, minced
10 mL (2 tsp.) oil
salt and pepper to taste

To prepare crust: in a bowl, combine dry ingredients and form a well at the center. Add water to oil and pour over dry ingredients. Mix until ingredients are moist. In a 20-cm (8-in.) pie plate, spread pastry evenly with fingers.

To prepare filling: wash spinach; drain lightly, place into saucepan, and cook 5 minutes only. Drain and chop finely; drain again. Sauté onion in oil for a few minutes until transparent. Add to spinach.

In a blender or food processor blend eggs and tofu. Add nutmeg, salt, and pepper to taste. Pour mixture over spinach, mix, and check seasoning. Pour onto pastry.

Bake about 30 minutes in a 190°C (375°F) oven, or until quiche is set. Serve with Fresh Tomato Coulis (see recipe index) or another home-made tomato sauce. Makes 8 small portions.

Each portion provides

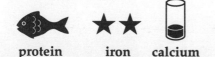

protein   iron   calcium

Salmon and Broccoli Quiche

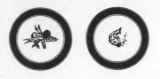

1 pie crust baked for 5 minutes
180 g (6 oz.) fresh or canned salmon
175 mL (¾ cup) cottage cheese
45 mL (3 tbsp.) cheddar cheese, shredded
2 eggs
250 mL (1 cup) milk
300 mL (1¼ cups) broccoli florets
dash of nutmeg

Mix salmon and cottage cheese and spread on half-baked pie crust. Add broccoli. Beat eggs; add milk and nutmeg and pour over mixture. Sprinkle with cheddar cheese.

Bake about 45 minutes in a 190°C (375°F) oven, or until pie is evenly set and golden. Makes 6 to 8 portions.

Each portion provides

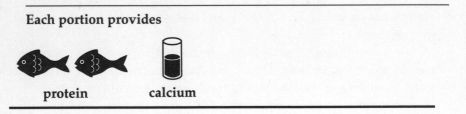

protein   calcium

Salmon Soufflé

439 g (15½ oz.) can salmon
45 mL (3 tbsp.) butter
60 mL (4 tbsp.) flour
250 mL (1 cup) liquid or (150 mL milk plus liquid from salmon)
3 egg yolks, beaten
3 egg whites, beaten to form stiff peaks
pepper to taste

Drain salmon and flake. Melt butter and add flour and salmon liquid. Heat until thick, stirring constantly. Add pepper. Allow to cool slightly. Add yolks and salmon, then fold in whites.

Pour into an ungreased baking pan. Place pan into another baking pan filled with 2.5 cm (1 in.) water. Bake 45 minutes in 180°C (350°F) oven. Makes 10 portions.

Each portion provides

proteins   calcium

Vegetable Pie

1 whole wheat pie crust, baked 5 minutes
375 mL (1½ cups) zucchini, thinly sliced
375 mL (1½ cups) fresh mushrooms, cut into pieces
250 mL (1 cup) fresh broccoli, cut into small pieces
15 mL (1 tbsp.) butter
15 mL (1 tbsp.) oil
250 mL (1 cup) milk
30 mL (2 tbsp.) whole wheat flour
3 eggs
120 g (1 cup) cheese, shredded
salt and pepper to taste
sesame seeds

In a large skillet or wok, brown vegetables in butter and oil a few minutes until slightly tender. Place on pie crust.

In a blender or food processor, blend milk, flour, eggs, and cheese until smooth. Season to taste with salt and pepper. Pour over vegetables. Sprinkle with sesame seeds.

Bake 20 to 30 minutes in a 220°C (425°F) oven, or until pie is set. Makes 6 to 8 small portions.

Each portion provides

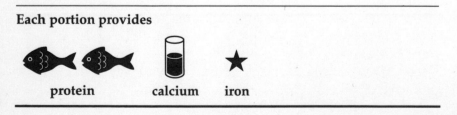

protein   calcium   iron

Happy Endings

Fruit Kabob

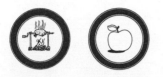

1 banana, cut into 4 pieces
1 pineapple slice, cut into 4 pieces
1 orange, divided into sections
1 apple, cut into wedges
1 peach, cut into pieces
4 prunes, pitted
plain yogurt (optional)
chopped nuts or grated coconut, to taste

Fruit Marinade
125 mL (½ cup) unsweetened orange juice
125 mL (½ cup) pineapple juice
30 mL (2 tbsp.) lemon juice
30 mL (2 tbsp.) honey
2 mL (½ tsp.) cinnamon
2 mL (½ tsp.) ginger

In a bowl, mix marinade ingredients. Add fruits and marinate 1 hour. Drain fruits and thread alternately onto 4 skewers. Set under the broiler 7 to 10 minutes.

Serve kabobs dipped in marinade or plain yogurt, coated with chopped nuts or grilled coconut. Makes 4 portions.

Each portion provides

vitamin C

Miracle Compote

 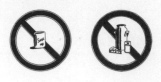

6 large apples, unpeeled
250 mL (1 cup) prunes, pitted
125 mL ($\frac{1}{2}$ cup) apple juice

Cut apples into wedges; core and stem. Place all ingredients into a large saucepan and simmer over medium heat for about 30 minutes or until apples are tender.

Remove from heat and pour half of mixture into blender or food processor, purée, and pour into a bowl. Repeat for the other half. Allow to cool and keep refrigerated until served. Makes about 500 mL (2 cups) or 10 servings.

Each portion provides

fiber

Spring Compote

 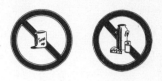

500 mL (2 cups) fresh rhubarb
500 mL (2 cups) apples
125 mL (½ cup) raisins
75 mL (5 tbsp.) water
dash of cinnamon

Cut rhubarb into pieces 5 cm (2 in.) long. Peel and cut apples into wedges; core. Place all ingredients into a saucepan, except for cinnamon, and simmer until apples are tender. Purée mixture in blender or food processor. Add cinnamon to taste. Allow to cool and keep refrigerated until served. Makes about 500 mL (2 cups) or 10 servings.

Each portion provides

fiber

Blueberry Crunch

500 mL (2 cups) fresh or frozen blueberries, unsweetened
4 apples, peeled, cored, and cut into pieces
250 mL (1 cup) whole wheat flour
75 mL (5 tbsp.) brown sugar
5 mL (1 tsp.) baking powder
2 mL ($\frac{1}{2}$ tsp.) salt
1 egg, beaten
2 mL ($\frac{1}{2}$ tsp.) cinnamon

Place blueberries and apples into a square Pyrex dish; mix lightly. In another bowl, combine flour, brown sugar, baking powder, and salt. Add beaten egg and stir until ingredients are moist. Pour mixture onto fruits and sprinkle generously with cinnamon.

Bake 30 minutes in a 190°C (375°F) oven. Makes 8 portions.

Each portion provides

protein

Apple and Almond Custard

75 mL (⅓ cup) almonds, not blanched
1 shredded wheat biscuit
4 medium apples, peeled and thinly sliced
75 mL (⅓ cup) raisins
zest of half an orange and half a lemon
250 mL (1 cup) milk
2 eggs
1 banana

In a blender or food processor, grind the almonds and the shredded wheat biscuit.

Grease baking plate; sprinkle bottom with a third of the almond crumbs; add 1 layer apples, 1 layer raisins and zest; start over and finish with a layer of almond crumbs.

In a blender or food processor blend milk, eggs, and banana, pour onto fruits. Bake about 45 minutes in a 180°C (350°F) oven or until custard is set and golden. Makes 8 portions.

This sugarless, high-protein dessert can complement a light meal.

Each portion provides

protein

Carob Cake

375 mL ($1\frac{1}{2}$ cups) whole wheat cake flour
125 mL ($\frac{1}{2}$ cup) brown sugar
45 mL (3 tbsp.) carob powder
5 mL (1 tsp.) baking soda
2 mL ($\frac{1}{2}$ tsp.) salt
250 mL (1 cup) water
90 mL (6 tbsp.) sunflower oil
15 mL (1 tbsp.) vinegar
5 mL (1 tsp.) vanilla

In a 20 x 20-cm (8 x 8-in.) cake pan combine all dry ingredients. Make a well at the center and add liquid ingredients. Stir until mixture is homogeneous.

Bake 30 to 35 minutes in 180°C (350°F) oven.

Serve hot with a creamed tofu sauce.

Each portion provides

fiber

Lemon and Cinnamon Cream of Wheat Cake

Cake
45 mL (3 tbsp.) butter
45 mL (3 tbsp.) brown sugar
2 eggs
250 mL (1 cup) fortified cream of wheat
125 mL (½ cup) ground almonds
5 mL (1 tsp.) cinnamon
2 mL (½ tsp.) vanilla

Syrup
250 mL (1 cup) water
45 mL (3 tbsp.) brown sugar
30 mL (2 tbsp.) lemon juice
zest from half a lemon

Cream butter and brown sugar until mixture is smooth and sugar is dissolved. Add eggs and beat. Stir in all other ingredients and mix well. Pour into a greased 20 x 20-cm (8 x 8-in.) cake pan. Bake 40 to 50 minutes in a 180°C (350°F) oven. Cake is ready when a knife inserted into center comes out clean. Let stand 10 minutes, then coat with hot syrup.

Syrup: in a small saucepan bring all ingredients to a boil; simmer for 10 minutes. Pour over warm cake and let stand at least 30 minutes before serving.

Cut into 5-cm (2-in.) squares and serve with a dollop of plain yogurt (optional). Makes 16 squares.

Each square provides

iron

Prune Juice Jelly

 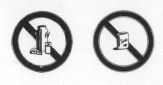

1 envelope gelatin, unflavored
45 mL (3 tbsp.) orange juice
250 mL (1 cup) prune juice
125 mL (½ cup) orange juice
1 small banana

In a medium bowl, sprinkle gelatin over 45 mL (3 tbsp.) orange juice and allow to dissolve. Bring prune juice to a boil. In the meantime, purée rest of orange juice and banana in a blender.

Pour hot prune juice over thickened gelatin and stir well to dissolve. Add orange/banana mixture and stir. Refrigerate about 2 hours. Serve plain or with a dollop of vanilla yogurt. Makes 6 small portions.

Each portion provides

iron

Sunny Date and Apricot Jelly

 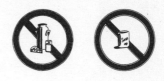

125 mL (½ cup) dried apricots, chopped
125 mL (½ cup) dates, chopped
175 mL (⅔ cup) water
45 mL (3 tbsp.) water
1 envelope gelatin, unflavored
175 mL (⅔ cup) concentrated white grape juice
5 mL (1 tsp.) vanilla

Over low heat, simmer apricots and dates in water. In a large bowl, sprinkle gelatin over 45 mL (3 tbsp.) water and let sit about 10 minutes.

Remove dried fruits and water from heat, purée in a blender or food processor, pour over gelatin and stir until dissolved. Add cold grape juice and vanilla and stir. Pour into individual dessert cups and allow to set a few hours in the refrigerator. Serve with a dollop of plain yogurt (optional). Makes 6 small servings.

Each portion provides

iron   vitamin A

Banana and Almond Muffins

125 mL ($\frac{1}{2}$ cup) ground oatmeal
125 mL ($\frac{1}{2}$ cup) oat bran
125 mL ($\frac{1}{2}$ cup) potato starch
45 mL (3 tbsp.) rice flour
45 mL (3 tbsp.) soy flour
2 mL ($\frac{1}{2}$ tsp.) nutmeg
2 mL ($\frac{1}{2}$ tsp.) salt
5 mL (1 tsp.) baking soda
2 ripe bananas, puréed
15 mL (1 tsp.) white vinegar
75 mL (5 tbsp.) sunflower oil
75 mL (5 tbsp.) maple syrup or honey
15 mL (1 tbsp.) almond extract
250 mL (1 cup) almond milk (see page 000)

In a bowl, place all dry ingredients, mix well. In a blender or food processor, purée bananas and add rest of liquid ingredients. Combine with dry ingredients and stir until moistened. Pour into greased muffin pan.

Bake 20 minutes at 190°C (375°F). Makes 12 medium muffins.

Each muffin provides

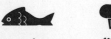

proteins   fiber

Orange Muffins

1 orange, not peeled, cut into wedges
125 mL ($\frac{1}{2}$ cup) orange juice
125 mL ($\frac{1}{2}$ cup) dates, chopped
1 egg
45 mL (3 tbsp.) honey
250 mL (1 cup) whole wheat cake flour
500 mL (2 cups) iron-fortified infant cereal
10 mL (2 tsp.) baking powder
2 mL ($\frac{1}{2}$ tsp.) salt

In a blender or food processor, purée orange. Add juice, chopped dates, egg, oil, and honey and stir well. In a large bowl, combine dry ingredients. Add liquids to dry ingredients and stir until moistened. Pour mixture into well greased muffin pans.

Bake about 15 minutes at 200°C (400°F). Makes 12 muffins.

Each muffin provides

iron

Bran Muffins

250 mL (1 cup) whole wheat flour
250 mL (1 cup) natural wheat bran
45 mL (3 tbsp.) brown sugar
7 mL (1½ tsp.) baking powder
2 mL (½ tsp.) baking soda
2 mL (½ tsp.) salt
125 mL (½ cup) orange juice, unsweetened
125 mL (½ cup) prune nectar, unsweetened
2 eggs

In a large bowl, combine dry ingredients; in another bowl mix all liquid ingredients. Combine liquid ingredients with dry ingredients until moistened. Pour into greased muffin pans.

Bake 45 to 50 minutes at 180°C (350°F). Makes 12 medium muffins.

Each muffin provides

fiber

Frozen Oranges

4 oranges
125 mL (½ cup) plain yogurt
15 mL (1 tbsp.) honey

Halve oranges, scoop out pulp, reserve for use (remove white central membrane). Freeze orange shells.

Purée yogurt, honey, and orange pulp and freeze 1 hour, then beat with whisk or mixer. Stuff orange shells with mixture, wrap, and return to freezer. Remove from freezer half an hour before serving. Makes 4 to 8 portions.

Each portion provides

vitamin C

Orange Ice Cream

1 385-mL (14-oz.) can evaporated milk
250 mL (1 cup) concentrated orange juice (unfrozen)
30 mL (2 tbsp.) white sugar or honey

Pour evaporated milk into a metal bowl and freeze until crystals start forming around the edges. With mixer, beat milk until stiff peaks form (about 5 minutes). Add orange juice and sugar. (At this point it can be served as Orange Mousse or Orange Whipped Cream.)

Return to freezer for 1½ to 2 hours or until mixture is almost set. Serve. For a smoother consistency, beat again and return to freezer until ice cream is firm. Makes 10 portions.

Serve with orange slices.

Each serving contains 40 times more vitamin C and 50 percent less fat than regular vanilla ice cream.

Each portion provides

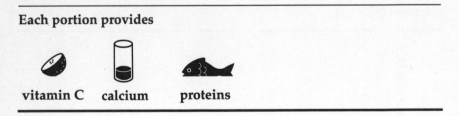

vitamin C   calcium   proteins

Barbecued Apple on a Stick

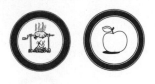

1 apple
1 stick

Cut a Y-shaped stick from a tree branch. Wedge apple (with peel) firmly into "Y." Grill over camp fire or barbecue.

With supervision, children can cook the apples themselves. Apples should be firmly positioned on the stick since they soften during cooking and may fall into the fire.

Each apple provides

fiber

Other Food Ideas

Almond and Sesame Milk

125 mL (½ cup) almonds, blanched
125 mL (½ cup) sesame seeds
dash of salt
15 mL (1 tbsp.) oil
15 to 30 mL (1 to 2 tbsp.) honey
1 L (4 cups) boiling water

Place all ingredients in blender except for water. Add boiling water gradually while blending until smooth. Taste, and adjust honey. Filter through a cheese cloth; refrigerate liquid and keep residue for cookies. Makes 1 liter (4 cups).

A 250 mL (1 cup) portion provides

proteins   calcium

Concentrated Almond Milk

100 g (⅔ cup) almonds, blanched
15 mL (1 tbsp.) vegetable oil
15 mL (1 tbsp.) honey or maple syrup
125 mL (½ cup) water

In a blender or food processor finely grind almonds. Add all other ingredients and blend until homogeneous. Makes 250 mL (1 cup).

A 250 mL (1 cup) portion provides

calcium   iron   protein

Tahini Salad Dressing

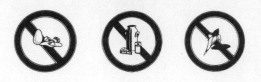

125 mL (½ cup) water
125 mL (½ cup) tahini
15 mL (1 tbsp.) fresh lemon juice
1 clove garlic, minced
dash thyme
dash basil

Place all ingredients into blender and blend for about 1 minute. Makes 250 mL (1 cup).

Tastier when prepared a day in advance. Keeps 2 weeks in refrigerator.

Lean Salad Dressing

45 mL (3 tbsp.) low fat yogurt
5 mL (1 tsp.) vinegar
5 mL (1 tsp.) prepared mustard
1 mL ($\frac{1}{4}$ tsp.) salt
1 mL ($\frac{1}{4}$ tsp.) pepper

Mix all ingredients well. Makes 4 portions of 15 mL (1 tbsp.).

Mayonnaise contains 9 times more calories than this dressing.

Appendix A

Nutrient Tables

Dairy Products		
cheese (hard)	30 g	1 oz.
cottage cheese	50 mL	¼ cup
milk, all types	125 mL	½ cup
skim milk powder	15 mL	1 tbsp.
yogurt	125 mL	½ cup
Fats		
butter	5 mL	1 tsp.
oils, all types	5 mL	1 tsp.
Fish		
canned, all types	30 g	1 oz.
Fruits		
juices	125 mL	½ cup
whole	50 mL	¼ cup
Legumes		
cooked, all types	50 mL	¼ cup
Pasta and Grains		
pasta	90 mL	6 tbsp.
oatmeal, rice, etc	90 mL	6 tbsp.
Seeds and Nuts		
all types	15 mL	1 tbsp.
peanut butter	15 mL	1 tbsp.
Vegetables		
cooked, all types	50 mL	¼ cup
Other		
bran	15 mL	1 tbsp.
cocoa	15 mL	1 tbsp.
molasses	15 mL	1 tbsp.
tofu	30 g	1 oz.
wheat germ	15 mL	1 tbsp.
yeast	5 mL	1 tsp.

VITAMIN A
(retinol or beta-carotene)

Functions

- important for vision, especially night vision
- helps maintain healthy body tissues
- performs in the growth of bones and resistance against infections

Best Sources:

ANIMAL (as retinol)	IU	PLANT (as beta-carotene)	IU
beef liver	16,020	carrots, cooked	1016
lamb liver	11,835	spinach, cooked	2910
veal liver	9800	turnip greens, cooked	1830
turkey liver	5251	squash, cooked	1720
pork liver	4472	mango	1580
chicken liver	3690	beet greens, cooked	1480
1 large egg yolk	313	cantaloupe	1090
cheddar cheese	300	papaya	1020
goat's milk	240	1 apricot	960
2% milk	186	broccoli, cooked	830
whole milk	176	tomato juice	780
butter	127	romaine lettuce	530
		2 dried apricots	420
		½ tomato	410
		2 asparagus	270
		watermelon	190

For quantities see page 186.

Risk of Deficiency: Young children usually consume adequate vitamin A.

Overdose: Severe poisoning has been found in children regularly taking more than 4000 ER (13,000 IU) per day as retinol. Children who consume too many foods rich in beta-carotene display a harmless orange skin coloration that disappears when intake is back to normal.

Vulnerability: Cooking has no affect, but drying can cause losses.

Warning: Frequent use of mineral oil as a laxative prevents absorption of vitamin A.

Recommended Nutrient Intakes:

2–3 years: 1320 IU

4–6 years: 1665 IU

Available supplements: See Appendix B

THIAMINE
(vitamin B_1)

Functions
- transforms foods into energy and fat
- allows rapid use of muscular energy
- regulates nervous system

Best Sources:

ANIMAL	mg	PLANT	mg
pork	0.32	Torula yeast	0.42
ham	0.14	sunflower seeds	0.14
pork liver	0.10	wheat germ	0.10
soy beans	0.08	½ orange	0.09
plain yogurt	0.10	bran	0.08
goat's milk	0.10	whole wheat	
herring	0.05	bread	0.08
whole/2%/skim milk	0.05	1 egg	0.04
lamb	0.04	oatmeal	0.06
Boston blue fish	0.03	brown rice	0.06
lake trout	0.03	2 fresh asparagus	0.05
beef	0.02	lentils	0.04
		spinach, cooked	0.03
		broccoli	0.03
		sesame seeds	0.01

For quantities see page 186.

Risk of Deficiency: Uncommon in young children. Beriberi occurs in countries w..ere refined rice is a major part of diet.

Overdose: Can prevent absorption of other B-complex vitamins.

Vulnerability: Boiling, high temperatures, and alkaline mediums destroy thiamine.

Complement: Works with magnesium in the process of energy transformation.

Recommended Nutrient Intakes:
2–3 years: 0.6 mg/day
4–6 years: 0.7 mg/day

Available supplements: See Appendix B

RIBOFLAVIN
(vitamin B$_2$)

Functions

- required for transformation of proteins, fats, and sugars into energy
- essential for healthy skin, mucous membranes, and cornea

Risk of Deficiency: Vegan or macrobiotic children.

Overdose: No documented danger of overdose.

Vulnerability: Destroyed by light and cooking in water.

Recommended Nutrient Intakes:

2–3 years: 0.7 mg/day

4–6 years: 0.9 mg/day

Available supplements: See Appendix B

Best Sources

ANIMAL	mg	PLANT	mg
beef kidneys	1.37	Torula yeast	0.07
pork liver	1.31	fortified cereal	0.18–0.39
beef liver	1.26	fortified noodles,	
veal liver	1.25	cooked	0.20
beef heart	0.36	raw mushrooms	0.09
yogurt 2%	0.30	broccoli, cooked	0.07
frozen milk	0.21	rice infant cereal	0.06
skim milk	0.18	wheat germ	0.06
ice cream	0.17	2 asparagus, cooked	0.05
Camembert cheese	0.14	spinach, cooked	0.05
cottage cheese	0.12	enriched white bread	0.05
		split peas	0.05
		2 Brussels sprouts	0.04
		pinto beans	0.04
		whole wheat bread	0.04
		soy beans	0.03
		lentils	0.02

For quantities see page 186.

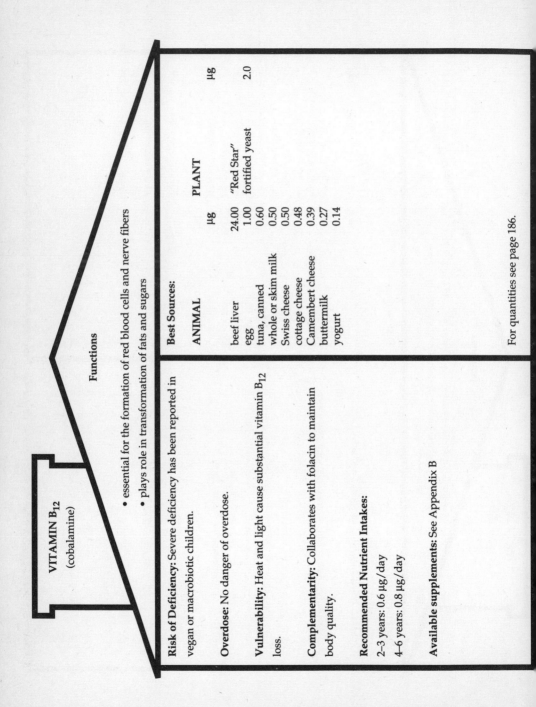

VITAMIN B₁₂
(cobalamine)

Functions

- essential for the formation of red blood cells and nerve fibers
- plays role in transformation of fats and sugars

Best Sources:

ANIMAL	μg	PLANT	μg
beef liver	24.00	"Red Star" fortified yeast	2.0
egg	1.00		
tuna, canned	0.60		
whole or skim milk	0.50		
Swiss cheese	0.50		
cottage cheese	0.48		
Camembert cheese	0.39		
buttermilk	0.27		
yogurt	0.14		

Risk of Deficiency: Severe deficiency has been reported in vegan or macrobiotic children.

Overdose: No danger of overdose.

Vulnerability: Heat and light cause substantial vitamin B₁₂ loss.

Complementarity: Collaborates with folacin to maintain body quality.

Recommended Nutrient Intakes:

2–3 years: 0.6 μg/day
4–6 years: 0.8 μg/day

Available supplements: See Appendix B

For quantities see page 186.

FOLACIN
(folic acid)

Functions

- required for the formation of red blood cells
- plays essential role in numerous reactions

Best Sources:

ANIMAL	µg	PLANT	µg
beef liver	90	2 brussels sprouts	65
fresh oysters	70	soy beans	94
1 large egg	50	orange juice, fresh	82
plain yogurt	14	Torula yeast	80
whole and skim milk	7	chick peas	50
goat's milk	2	kidney beans	49
		orange ($\frac{1}{2}$)	42
		spinach, cooked	39
		romaine lettuce	39
		beets , cooked	33
		sweet potato	28
		asparagus	21
		broccoli, cooked	18
		wheat germ	16
		whole wheat bread	15
		peanut butter	13
		cantaloupe	10

For quantities see page 186.

Risk of Deficiency: Rare in young children.

Overdose: In 1984 Health and Welfare issued a warning against the abuse of folic acid and suggested a maximum does of 1 mg per day for adults.

Can interfere with B$_{12}$ and anticonvulsant drugs and reduce zinc absorption.

Vulnerability: Cooking in water, heat, and storage at room temperature results in loss of folic acids in foods.

Complementarity: Works with iron and vitamin B$_{12}$ to maintain good quality blood.

Recommended Nutrient Intakes:

2–3 years: 50 µg/day

4–6 years: 70 µg/day

Available supplements: See Appendix B

VITAMIN C
(ascorbic acid)

Functions

- maintains cell structure
- performs in numerous reactions in the body

Best Sources:

ANIMAL	mg	PLANT	mg
veal liver, cooked	11	orange juice, fresh	60
chicken liver, cooked	5	1/4 raw red pepper	38
		2 Brussels sprouts	35
		papaya	34
		1/2 orange	33
		broccoli, cooked	30
		kale, cooked	28
		1/4 grapefruit	27
		1/4 green pepper, raw	24
		strawberries	18
		1/2 tomato, raw	17
		tomato juice	16
		cauliflower, cooked	14
		cantaloupe	11
		raw cabbage, grated	9
		2 asparagus spears	8
		raspberries	6

For quantities see page 186.

Risk of Deficiency: Children consume 4 times the recommended amount of vitamin C. Children who regularly take megadoses may develop deficiency symptoms when they stop.

Overdose: Rare since kidneys eliminate any excess.

Vulnerability: Heat, cooking in water, and exposure to air cause vitamin C loss. However, vitamin C is particularly stable in fruits and citrus fruit juices.

Complementarity: Increases absorption of iron.

Recommended Nutrient Intakes:

2–3 years: 20 mg/day

4–6 years: 25 mg/day

Available supplements: See Appendix B

VITAMIN D
(cholecalciferol D_3
and ergocalciferol D_2)

Functions

- helps build and maintain healthy bones
- prevents rickets

At Risk of Deficiency: Breast-fed babies not exposed to sunlight and not receiving supplements, vegan, and macrobiotic children.

Overdose: Doses of 75 to 100 µg per day can retard growth. Excess vitamin D can accumulate in the body.

Vulnerability: Cooking and storage do not affect vitamin D.

Recommended Nutrient Intakes:

2–3 years: 5 µg/day
4–6 years: 5 µg/day

Available supplements: See Appendix B

Best Sources:

ANIMAL	µg	PLANT (no good sources)
cod liver oil	6.00	
whole milk, 2%, skim	1.25	
1 large egg yolk	0.70	
skim milk powder	0.61	
chicken liver	0.39	
beef liver	0.33	
pork liver	0.33	
butter	0.12	

Other sources

sunlight: 20 square cm (3 square in.) of skin exposed 3 hours to sunlight absorb 10 µg vitamin D.

For quantities see page 186.

VITAMIN E
(alpha-tocopherol)

Functions

- protects red blood cells
- required for healthy muscles
- prevents foods from going rancid

At Risk of Deficiency: Healthy children are not at risk as needs are relatively low and several common foods contain it.

Overdose: Some adults react to doses exceeding 200 or 300 mg per day. Children should not take such high doses.

Vulnerability: Vitamin E may be lost during refining, freezer storage, or in stale oils.

Complementarity: Vitamin E works with selenium.

Recommended Nutrient Intakes:

2–3 years: 4 mg/day; 6.0 IU

4–6 years: 5 mg/day; 7.5 IU

Available supplements: See Appendix B

Best Sources:

ANIMAL	IU	PLANT	IU
1 egg yolk	0.9	wheat germ oil	13.4
butter	0.3	sunflower oil	4.5
whole milk	0.3	cotton oil	4.5
		saffron oil	4.5
		palm oil	3.0
		rape oil	3.0
		wild blackberries	2.5
		wheat germ	1.9
		2 asparagus, cooked	1.8
		brown rice, cooked	1.6
		½ apple	1.3
		1 leek	1.2
		½ pear	0.9
		broccoli	0.9
		2 large Brussels sprouts	0.6

For quantities see page 186.

CALCIUM

Functions

- helps build and maintain strong bones and teeth
- assists normal nerve and muscle function and blood clotting

At Risk of Deficiency: Vegan and macrobiotic children as well as children suffering from lactose intolerance or allergy are at risk in some adults.

Overdose: Can contribute to the formation of calcium deposits.

Vulnerability: Cooking does not affect calcium level, but large intake of proteins and fiber limit its absorption.

Complementarity: Calcium works well with vitamin D and phosphorus.

Recommended Nutrient Intakes:
2–3 years: 550 mg/day
4–6 years: 600 mg/day

Available supplements: See Appendix B

Best Sources:

ANIMAL	mg	PLANT	mg
Swiss cheese	262	fortified soy milk	175
cheddar cheese	204	blackstrap molasses	137
plain yogurt	203	kale, cooked	72
whole goat's milk	172	cream of wheat, precooked	63
whole/2%/ skim milk	153–159	bok choy	50
butter milk	150	tofu	38
skim milk powder	113	mustard greens	36
sardines 2, canned	112	spinach, cooked	34
sockeye, salmon, canned with bones	78	chick peas	30
cottage cheese	22–31	broccoli, cooked	29
		soy beans	26
		sesame seeds	23
		10 almonds	23
		turnip, cooked	16
		Torula yeast	11

For quantities see page 186.

FLUORIDE

Function

- Fluoride taken in naturally rich or fluoridated water or in supplements helps build tooth enamel that resists cavities;
- Fluoride applied topically in fluoridated toothpaste neutralizes the acid environment of the mouth and prevents formation of cavities.

At risk of Deficiency: Children living in areas where water is not naturally or artificially fluoridated.

Overdose: White stains can occur on teeth in children who regularly receive doses exceeding 3 to 4 mg (ppm) per day.

Recommended Nutrient Intakes:
After the age of two, if the local water supply is not fluoridated, give 0.25 mg fluoride as a supplement.

Available supplements: See Appendix B

Best Sources:

	PLANT	mg
ANIMAL (no good sources)		
	tea	0.1–0.2

OTHER SOURCES

fluoridated water 0.09–0.15 mg
toothpaste 0.5–0.73 mg

For quantities see page 186.

IRON

Functions

- Essential for formation of hemoglobin, which transports oxygen in blood
- provides oxygen to muscles

At Risk of Deficiency: Children, especially those aged 18 mos. to 3 years.

Overdose: Iron supplements are the second highest cause of poisoning in children under 5. Some supplements can cause stomach pains.

Vulnerability: Water and cooking decrease the iron content of foods; always reserve cooking water for later use. Iron from animal sources is more easily absorbed and in larger quantities.

Complementarity: Iron is best absorbed when combined with a food rich in vitamin C.

Recommended Nutrient Intakes:

2–3 years: 6 mg/day

4–6 years: 8 mg/day

Available supplements: See Appendix B

Best Sources:

ANIMAL	mg	PLANT	mg
pork liver	8.70	prune juice	4.10
lamb liver	5.40	blackstrap molasses	3.20
veal liver	4.30	black beans	1.58
beef liver	2.70	chick peas	1.38
chicken liver	2.60	soy beans	0.98
3 small oysters	1.70	soy milk	0.90
sweet-water trout	1.50	Lima beans	0.86
pork	1.10	lentils	0.84
1 egg	1.10	spinach, cooked	0.84
lean beef	1.10	split peas	0.68
veal	1.00	Torula yeast	0.60
turkey	0.53	tofu	0.58
chicken	0.50	10 almonds	0.50
		2 dates	0.48
		wheat germ	0.41
		raisins	0.31
		strawberries	0.31
		oatmeal	0.29

For quantities see page 186.

MAGNESIUM

Functions

- Helps metabolize foods into energy
- Regulates nervous system

At Risk of Deficiency: There is little data on deficiency risks in young children.

Overdose: Dangers are still fairly unknown.

Vulnerability: Refining flours and cereals results in significant magnesium loss. Use whole grain flours.

Complementarity: Works with calcium, phosphorus, vitamin D, and the B vitamins.

Recommended Nutrient Intakes:

2–3 years: 50 mg/day

4–6 years: 65 mg/day

Available supplements: See Appendix B

Best Sources:

ANIMAL	mg	PLANT	mg
skim milk, buttermilk	17	soy beans	111
whole milk	16	black eye beans	78
skim milk powder	14	white beans	69
Cheddar cheese	14	tofu	67
ice cream	9	Lima beans	65
1 large egg	5	cashew nuts	50
		spinach, cooked	40
		beet leaves	33
		peanut butter	28
		almonds	28
		wheat germ	21
		cocoa	21
		brown rice	19
		oatmeal, cooked	17
		Torula yeast	4

For quantities see page 186.

POTASSIUM

Functions

- Maintains the balance of fluids inside cells
- Performs in several chemical reactions in the body

At Risk of Deficiency: Children who fast or have severe burns, prolonged fever, or chronic diarrhea, or use diuretics regularly can have considerable potassium loss.

Overdose: Excessive intake of supplements can be harmful to health.

Recommended Nutrient Intakes:
A minimum of 70 mg per day

Available supplements: See Appendix B

Best Sources:

ANIMAL	mg	PLANT	mg
milk powder	320	blackstrap molasses	585
plain yogurt	218	¼ cantaloupe	483
milk, whole, 2%, skim, buttermilk	196–214	¼ banana	324
ice cream	135	prune juice	318
beef	105	raisins	266
chicken	82	orange juice	262
1 egg	65	½ small potato	252
		musk squash	240
		pinto beans	226
		½ nectarine	203
		kidney beans	183
		¼ papaya	178
		soy beans	171
		Lima beans	151
		parsnip, cooked	118
		fresh peas	46

For quantities see page 186.

SODIUM

Functions

- Maintains fluid balance outside cells
- Performs in the transmission of nerve impulses and in muscular contractions

At Risk of Deficiency: Unlikely in our society.

Overdose: A high-salt diet can impede the proper treatment of hypertension.

Best Sources:

ANIMAL	mg	PROCESSED FOODS	mg
cottage cheese	192	2 slices bacon, grilled	884
cheddar cheese	186	smoked sausage	542
buttermilk	136	McDonald's hamburger	530
yogurt	73	$\frac{1}{4}$ large dill pickle	482
milk, whole,		McDonald's apple	
2%, skim	63–67	turnover	415
cod fillet, grilled	35	tomato juice, canned	256
fresh pork	18	smoked ham	227
		10 potato chips	200
PLANT		McDonald's chocolate	
		milkshake	165
carrots, cooked	10	1 stick frozen fish	158
$\frac{1}{4}$ fresh cucumber	3.0	ketchup	156
$\frac{1}{2}$ medium tomato	2.5	commercial salad dressing	152
$\frac{1}{2}$ baked potato	1.5	corn, canned	100
wax beans	0.8	wax beans, canned	94
fresh peas, cooked	0.6	carrots, canned	71
green peas, canned	63		

For quantities see page 186.

ZINC

Functions

- Important for the growth of body tissues
- Helps repair skin and prevents scarring

At Risk of Deficiency: Children with loss of appetite and may have low zinc intakes

Overdose: High dose supplements can compete with iron absorption.

Vulnerability: The body is better able to process zinc from animal sources than from plant sources.

Complementarity: Vitamin A

Recommended Nutrient Intakes:

2–3 years: 4 mg/day

4–6 years: 5 mg/day

Available Supplements: See Appendix B

Best Sources:

ANIMAL	mg	PLANT	mg
3 oysters	34.7	wheat germ	0.96
veal liver	1.84	peanut butter	0.50
beef	1.66	whole wheat bread	0.50
beef liver	1.53	brown rice	0.41
lamb	1.39	oatmeal	0.41
turkey, brown meat	1.31	lentils	0.40
crab	1.30	chick peas	0.40
pork	1.15	rye bread	0.40
chicken liver	1.01	bran	0.34
cheddar cheese	1.00	spinach, cooked	0.33
chicken, brown meat	0.85	split peas	0.28
turkey, white meat	0.64	green cabbage cooked	0.12
1 large yolk	0.50		
whole, 2%, skim milk	0.45		
ice cream	0.30		
chicken, white meat	0.25		

For quantities see page 186.

FIBER

Functions

- Increases bulk of foods in the digestive system, speeds up elimination, and reduces constipation
- Plays a role in satiety

At Risk of Deficiency: Young children who eat little or no fruits, vegetables and whole grains.

Overdose: Some vegan or macrobiotic children, who eat too many high-fiber foods do not eat enough calories to sustain normal growth; others can suffer from chronic diarrhea.

Vulnerability: The effects of cooking on fiber are little known.

Recommended Nutrient Intake:
No official recommendations; 15–20 g should be sufficient for a child.

Best Sources:

PLANT

	g		g
cereal products		*fruits*	
All-Bran	5.0	½ medium apple, with peel	2.0
oatmeal, cooked	3.5	½ pear, with peel	2.0
whole wheat bread	3.0	raspberries	1.8
natural bran	2.2	½ banana	1.5
whole wheat pasta	1.9	½ orange	1.2
brown rice	1.3	applesauce	1.0
½ shredded wheat biscuit	1.1	strawberries, pineapple	0.3
enriched white bread	0.8		
		vegetables	
legumes and nuts		green peas, broccoli	1.9
kidney beans	3.9	carrots	1.4
pinto beans	3.8	mushrooms raw,	
split peas	2.7	5 small	1.4
chick peas	2.4	zucchini	1.2
Lima beans	2.3	turnip	0.9
red lentils	1.3	½ small tomato	0.7
peanut butter	0.6	lettuce (Boston, Iceberg)	0.4
almonds, sliced	1.1		

For quantities see page 186.

PROTEIN

Functions

- Builds and repairs all body tissues
- Plays a role in the formation of antibodies and in the fight against infections

At Risk of Deficiency: Rare: young children usually consume 2 to 3 times the recommended amount of protein. Vegan and macrobiotic children must eat sufficient protein to develop normally.

Overdose: The body transforms excess protein into fat.

Vulnerability: Heat and cooking have little effect on proteins.

Complementarity: Animal proteins are complete. Plant protein is incomplete and should be combined with other foods during the same meal. For example: cereal with dairy products; legumes with cereal products; legumes with nuts or seeds.

Recommended Nutrient Intake:

2–3 years: 16 grams/day
4–6 years: 19 grams/day

Best Sources:

ANIMAL	mg	PLANT	mg
beef kidneys	10.0	peanut butter	4.40
turkey	9.3	soy beans	4.00
veal liver	9.0	chick peas	4.00
pork liver	9.0	lentils	3.20
tuna, canned	8.7	Lima beans	3.20
lean pork	8.3	whole wheat bread	3.00
chicken liver	8.0	tofu	2.50
beef	8.0	peanuts	2.40
beef liver	8.0	sunflower seeds	2.20
veal	8.0	oatmeal	1.70
salmon	8.0	wheat germ	1.50
lamb	7.8	nuts, chopped	1.50
chicken	7.0	sesame seeds	1.50
10 medium shrimp	7.0	cream of wheat	1.40
cheddar cheese	7.0	infant "high pro" cereal	0.83
1 large egg	6.0		
plain yogurt	6.0		
cottage cheese	6.0		
milk 2%, skim	4.5		
buttermilk	4.5		
goat's milk	4.5		
whole milk	4.0		

For quantities see page 186.

Vitamin and Mineral Supplements

	Vitamin A (IU)	Vitamin D (IU)	Vitamin C (mg)	Fluoride (mg)	Vitamin B1 (mg)	Vitamin B2 riboflavin (mg)	Niacin (mg)	Iron (mg)	Vitamin B6 (mg)	Vitamin B12 (µg)	Folate (mg)	Others
Bugs Bunny Complete Multivitamins (Miles) dosage: 1 tablet daily	5000	400	50		1.5	1.5	15	4	1	3	0.1	pantothenic acid: 10 mg, vitamin E: 10 IU, biotin: 30 mg, calcium: 125 mg, copper: 1 mg
Bugs Bunny Multivitamins (Miles) dosage: 1 tablet daily	5000	400	50		1.5	1.5	15	4	1	3	0.1	
Bugs Bunny Multivitamins with iron (Miles) dosage: 1 tablet daily	5000	400	50	1	1.5	1.5	15	4	1	3	0.1	
Centrum Junior Complete Vitamins and Minerals Chewable (Lederle) dosage: 1 tablet daily	5000	400	50	1	1.5	1.7	20	4	4	2	0.1	biotin: 30 mg, vitamin E: 10 IU, calcium: 162 mg, phosphorus: 125 mg, copper: 1 mg, iodine: 0.15 mg
Centrum Junior Regular Vitamins and Minerals Chewable (Lederle) dosage: 1 tablet daily	5000	400	50		1.5	1.7	20	4	4	2	0.1	pantothenic acid: 10 mg, calcium: 162 mg, phosphorus: 125 mg
Centrum Junior with Fluoride (Lederle) dosage: 1 tablet daily	5000	400	50		1.5	1.7	20	4	4	2	0.1	pantothenic acid: 10 mg, calcium: 162 mg, phosphorus: 125 mg

Product / dosage											Other
Children's Chewable Vita-Mints (Seroyal) dosage: 2 tablets daily	2000	200	50	1	0.5	2.5	2.5	1	5	0.2	vitamin E: 7.5 IU, biotin: 50 mcg, calcium: 20 mg, magnesium: 20 mg, zinc: 2.5 mg, manganese: 1 mg, copper: 0.25 mg, iodine: 0.035, bioflavonoides: 5 mg, rosehips 5 mg
Children's Chewable Vitamins (Vita Health) dosage: 1 tablet daily	5000	400	100	2	2	15	4	4	2		vitamin E: 10 IU
Children's Chewable Vitamins with Iron Vita-Health dosage: 1 tablet daily	5000	400	100	2	2	15	4	4	2		vitamin E: 10 IU, rosehips 10 mg
Children's Chewable Vitamins with Iron (Novopharm) dosage: 1 tablet daily	5000	400	50	1	1.5	15	4	4	1		pantothenic acid: 6 mg
Children's Chewable Vitamins with Iron and C (Vitapharm) dosage: 1 tablet daily	5000	400	100	1.5	1.2	10	5	6	1		vitamin E: 5 IU, pantothenic acid: 10 mg

	Vitamin A (IU)	Vitamin D (IU)	Vitamin C (mg)	Fluoride (mg)	Vitamin B1 (mg)	Vitamin B2 riboflavin (mg)	Niacin (mg)	Iron (mg)	Vitamin B6 (ug)	Vitamin B12 (mg)	Folate (mg)	Others
Cod Liver Oil (Vita Health) dosage: 5 ml daily	1250	100										
Cod Liver Oil (Swiss Herbal) dosage: 5 ml daily	1250	100										
Fer-in-Sol Drops (Mead Johnson) dosage: 0.3–0.6 ml/daily								0.6 ml = 15 mg				
Fer-in-Sol Syrop (Mead Johnson) dosage: 0–2 years/2.5–5 ml 0–6 years/5 ml								5 ml = 30 mg				
Fertinic Ferrous Gluconate Syrop (Desbergers) dosage: 5 ml/daily								35				
Flintstones Multiple Vitamins (Miles) dosage: 1 tablet daily	5000	400	50		1.5	1.5	15		1.10	3	0.1	

Product / dosage										
Flintstones Complete Multiple Vitamins Formula with Calcium, Iron, and Other Minerals (Miles) dosage: 1 tablet daily	5000	400	50	1.5	1.5	5	4	1.0	3	0.1	pantothenic acid: 10 mg, vitamin E: 10 IU, biotin: 30 mg, calcium: 160 mg, phosphorus: 125 mg, copper: 1 mg
Flintstones Multiple Vitamins with Extra C (Miles) dosage: 1 tablet daily	5000	400	250	1.5	1.5	15	4	1.0	3	0.1
Flintstones Multiple Vitamins with Iron (Miles) dosage: 1 tablet daily	5000	400	50	1.5	1.5	15	4	1.0	3	0.1
Garfield Chewable Multivitamins(Whitehall-Robins) dosage: 1 tablet daily	5000	400	75	1.5	1.5	15	4			
Garfield Chewable Multivitamins with Iron (Whitehall-Robins) dosage: 1 tablet daily	5000	400	75	1.5	1.5	15	4			
Glycobal Vitamin Tonic (Nabay) dosage: 1 teaspoon/daily				2.50	1.2	9.3		1.0			calcium: 75 mg, manganese: 20 mg, potassium: 60 mg, sodium: 100 mg

	Vitamin A (IU)	Vitamin D (IU)	Vitamin C (mg)	Fluoride (mg)	Vitamin B1 (mg)	Vitamin B2 riboflavin (mg)	Niacin (mg)	Iron (mg)	Vitamin B6 (ug)	Vitamin B12 (mg)	Folate (mg)	Others
Incremin with Iron (Lederle) dosage: 5 ml daily					4.5			30	25	5		
Infantol (Horner) dosage: 0.5 ml daily	1500	400	50		1.25	2.0	12.5		1.2			
Karidium (Lorvic Corp.) dosage: 1-4 years/4 drops				2.21								sodium chloride: 10 mg
Maxi-6 Liquid Multivitamin (Desbergers) dosage 1 teaspoon/daily	2500	400	40		0.8	0.9	11					
Natural Choice Vitamins and Minerals (Wampole) dosage: 1 tablet daily	5000	400	50		3	5	25	5	5	2	0.1	pantothenic acid: 15 mg, copper: 1 mg
Pardec Liquid (Parke Davis) dosage: 5 ml daily	5000	400	50		3	3	20		5	2		
Pardec Tablets (Parke Davis) dosage: 1 tablet daily	10 000	400			4.5	7.5	45	6	2	10		pantothenic acid: 7.5 mg, vitamin E: 10 IU, sodium ascorbate: 150 mg

Chewable Parametes for Children
(Whitehall-Robins)
dosage:
1 tablet daily

5000	400	75	1.5	1.5	15			

Chewable Parametes for Children with Iron
(Whitehall-Robins)
dosage:
1 tablet daily

5000	400	75	1.5	1.5	15	4		

Parametes Syrop
(Whitehall-Robins)
dosage:
5 ml daily

2500	200	20	1	1	5	4	2	0.6

Pediatri-Vite Liquid
(Seroyal Canada Inc.)
dosage:
1 teaspoon daily

1666	166	50	0.8	0.8	3.3	3.3	1.0	8.3	66 mcg

vitamin E: 10 IU, biotin: 66.5, pantothenic acid: 1.65 mg, calcium: 25 mg, potassium: 8.3 mg, magnesium: 4.17 mg, zinc: 3.3 mg, manganese: 0.8 mg, copper: 0.5 mg, iodine: 25 mcg, Molybdenium 83 mcg, vanadium: 83 mcg, chrome: 33 mcg, selenium: 33 mcg, choline: 10 mg, inositol: 0.8 mg

Poly-Vi-Flor Drops
(Mead Johnson)
dosage:
0.6 ml

1500	400	30	0.5	0.6	4			

Vitamin	Vitamin A (IU)	Vitamin D (IU)	Fluoride	Vitamin C (mg)	Vitamin (mg)	Vitamin B1 (mg)	Vitamin B2 riboflavin (mg)	Niacin (mg)	Iron (mg)	Vitamin B6 (mg)	Vitamin B12 (mg)	Folate (mg)	Others
Poly-Vi-Flor Tablets (Mead Johnson) dosage: 1 tablet daily	4000	400		75	1	1.2	1.5	15					
Poly-Vi-Sol (Mead Johnson) dosage: 0.6 ml	1500	400		30		0.5	0.6	4					
Poly-Vi-Sol (Mead Johnson) dosage: 1 tablet daily	4000	400		75		1.2	1.5	15					
Sesame Street Vitamins (McNeil) dosage: 1 tablet daily mg	5000	400		60		1.5	1.7	20		6	2	0.4	pantothenic acid: 10 mg, vitamin E: 15 IU, biotin: 30
Sesame Street Vitamins and Minerals (McNeil) dosage: 1 tablet daily	5000	400		60		1.5	1.7	20	4	6	2	0.4	pantothenic acid: 10 mg, vitamin E: 15 IU, biotin: 30 mg, iodine: 0.15 mg, copper: 2 mg
Smiles (Wampole) dosage: 1 tablet daily	5000	400		50		2	1.5	15		3	1.5	0.1	pantothenic acid: 10 mg, biotin: 30 ug, vitamin E: 30 ug, vitamin E: 10 IU
Smiles with Iron (Wampole) dosage: 1 tablet daily	5000	400		50		2	1.5	15	4	3	1.5	0.1	pantothenic acid: 10 mg, biotin: 15 ug

Product / dosage										
Special Formulated Chewable Children's Multi Vits (Hall) dosage: 1 tablet daily	3000	400	40	0.8	0.8	8	8	4	0.08	0.2
Tri-Vi-Flor (Mead Johnson) dosage: 0.6 ml	1500	400	30	0.5						
Tri-Vi-Flor (Mead Johnson) dosage: 1 tablet	4000	400	75	1						
Tri-Vi-Sol with Fluoride (Mead Johnson) dosage: 0.6 ml	1500	400	30	0.25						
Tri-Vi-Sol (Mead Johnson) dosage: 0.6 ml	1500	400	30							
Zoo Chews (Children's Chewables) (Hall) dosage: 1 tablet daily	5000	400	50	1.5	1.7	15	4	3	1	0.1
Zoo Chews with Iron (Children's Chewables) (Hall) dosage: 1 tablet daily	5000	400	50	1.5	1.7	15	15	3	1	0.1

Fortified Soy Milk Recipe

HOMEMADE SOY MILK from soy beans or powder does not contain enough calories or calcium to support normal growth in the vegan or microbiotic child.

To remedy these deficiencies, you must add to each 250 mL (1 cup) cooled soy milk:

5 mL (1 tsp.) corn or sunflower oil
10 mL (2 tsp.) brown sugar
10 mL (2 tsp.) calcium lactate powder (available in pharmacies or health food stores).

You may replace the calcium lactate with liquid calcium or calcium carbonate if the child has a lactose intolerance.

To improve the milk's taste, you can add a drop of vanilla or a dash of nutmeg; you may also add fortified soy milk to soups, desserts, or other dishes.

Soy milk infant formulas are already fortified.

Appendix D

Recommendations for Preventing and Treating Child Obesity in the United States*

RECOMMENDATIONS FOR IMPROVING THE OVERALL WELL-BEING OF CHILDREN

Create a Cabinet-Level Position on the Child and Family

Because of the unique vulnerability of children and the relationship of so many childhood problems to the health of the family, a cabinet-level position focusing on the well-being of the child and family is warranted. This individual could coordinate and plan a range of policies and programs to put children and families first.

Provide More Economic and Social Support for Low-Income Children

Obesity is more common among the very rich and the very poor. Child obesity rates increase in areas struck by economic hardship. Policies that support a thriving middle class would be likely to contribute to decreasing the prevalence and severity of obesity in children.

Beyond economic support, more services should be provided to low-income children (e.g., making safe recreational activities and parks available in low-income areas, ensuring through supplemental food programs that fruits, vegetables, grains, and other low-fat foods are consistently available; and providing economic and social support to enable parents to be more available to their children). Targeting the family is important because insufficient parental nurturing leaves children at risk of emotional overeating. Ineffective limit-setting may lead children to develop poor diet and exercise patterns.

Implement a National Plan for High-Quality After-School Care and Day Care

Our country has not effectively addressed the day care needs of children of working parents. Many children are home with no supervision

*Laurel Millin, Director, Center for Child and Adolescent Obesity, text published in the Journal of the American Dietetic Association, March 1993, Page 266

and with food and television as their only sources of companionship and recreation. Alternatives need to be developed, such as after-school care that includes physical activity, healthful snacks, and social interaction, all of which contribute to the prevention of obesity in children.

Mandate Health-Promoting Environments in Public Schools

Require daily physical education classes that teach endurance and lifetime physical activity skills. Modify school food programs so that nutrients are consistent with National Cholesterol Education Program guidelines. Implement a broad health education curriculum that teaches children to care for their emotional and physical well-being.

Create an Advisory Committee on Children and Nutrition

Currently, there is no institutional mechanism for identifying and approaching nutrition problems affecting large population segments. An advisory committee on children and nutrition could develop recommendations to ensure that the young are well-nourished and that nutrition problems are effectively addressed. The committee could hold a White House Conference on Food and Nutrition (the first since 1968) to develop national recommendations for nutrition policy, including children's issues such as obesity and hunger.

RECOMMENDATIONS TO IMPROVE THE AVAILABILITY, ACCESSIBILITY, AND EFFECTIVENESS OF CHILD OBESITY SERVICES

Extend Coverage by Health Insurers to Family-Based Child Obesity Services

Few health insurers cover child obesity services. As a result, few obese children receive effective care. For all but the most economically advantaged families, family-based child obesity care is a financial hardship or an economic impossibility. Most children are denied this safe, effective care because of economic factors.

The recent rise in the prevalence of severity of obesity in the young portends notable increases in health-care costs as this generation of children reaches adulthood and experiences increased rates of diabetes, cardiovascular disease, stroke, pulmonary problems, orthopedic problems, cancer, and other conditions. There is an important need to make these services widely available to children from families from all economic levels so that this trend of increasing prevalence of obesity in the young does not continue.

Our nation must recognize the financial impact of child obesity on national health care costs and to shape reimbursement policies of health insurers accordingly. We cannot afford to make economic disadvantage a barrier to receiving effective care for child and adolescent obesity.

Designate Increased Funding for Training in Child Obesity

Child obesity care providers work within an interdisciplinary team but need basic competencies in a range of areas pertinent to child obesity, including assessing family functioning, identifying sexual and physical abuse, and providing nutritional counselling. Providers require specialized child obesity training to develop these skills.

Comprehensive clinical training in child and adolescent obesity has been almost completely unavailable. UCSF has developed self-study comprehensive child obesity training, but participants are almost exclusively providers serving middle- and upper-income classes rather than those who serve the economically disadvantaged children who are most in need.

The shortage of trained child obesity specialists is a well-recognized barrier to addressing the problem of child obesity. Support for a broad range of training activities in child obesity, from university fellowships to courses for undergraduate students to professional continuing education courses, is needed.

Designate increased research funding for the prevention and treatment of child obesity

The National Institutes for Health Initiative on Obesity has provided funding for obesity research; however, more funding designated for research related to child and adolescent obesity is needed. A high priority should be given to research that has immediate practical applications to the prevention and treatment of obesity in the young. Research funding is also needed for studies targeting groups at greater risk of obesity, particularly the handicapped and ethnocultural groups such as blacks, Hispanics, and Native Americans.

Bibliography

PART ONE

The Preschooler's Eating Habits

Albertson, A. M., et al. "Nutrient Intakes of 2–10-year-old American Children; 10-year Trends." *Journal of the American Dietetic Association* 92 (1992): 1492–1496.

Caliendo, M. A., et al. "Nutritional Status of Preschool Children." *Journal of the American Dietetic Association* 71 (1977): 21–26.

Chery, A., et al. "Portion Size of Common Foods Eaten by Young Children." *Journal of the Canadian Dietetic Association* 45 (1984): 230–233.

Leung, M., et al. "Dietary Intakes of Preschoolers." *Journal of the American Dietetic Association* 84 (1984): 551–554.

Schumilas, T. M., et al. "Family Characteristics and Dietary Intake of Preschool Children." *Journal of the Canadian Dietetic Association* 45 (1984): 119–127.

Williams, S., et al. "Contribution of Foodservice Programs in Preschool Centers to Children's Nutritional Needs." *Journal of the American Dietetic Association* 71 (1977): 610–613.

Your Child's Nutritional Needs

Birch, L. L., et al. "The Variability of Young Children's Energy Intake." *New England Journal of Medicine* (January 24, 1991): 232–235.

Chery, A., and Sabry, J. "Portion Size of Common Foods Eaten by Young Children."*Journal of the Canadian Dietetic Association* 45 (1984): 230–233.

Endres, J. B., and Rockwell, J. *Food, Nutrition and the Young Child*. St-Louis: Mosby, 1980.

Forbes, G. "Children and Food; Order Amid Chaos." *New England Journal of Medicine* (January 24, 1991): 262–263.

Health and Welfare Canada; "Report of the Scientific Review Committee." Ottawa, 1990.

Network of the Federal/Provincial/Territorial Group on Nutrition and the National Institute of Nutrition. " Promoting Nutritional Health during the Preschool Years: Canadian Guidelines." Ottawa, 1989.

Instinct Versus Needs

Birch, L. L., et al. "Caloric Compensation and Sensory Specific Satiety: Evidence for Self-regulation of Food Intake by Young Children." *Appetite* 7 (1986): 323–331.

Davis, M. Clara. "Self Selection of Diet by Newly Weaned Infants." *American Journal of Disease in Childhood* 36 (1928): 651–679.

———. "Results of the Self Selection of Diets by Young Children." *Canadian Medical Association Journal* 41 (1939): 257–261.

———. "Self Selection of Food by Children." *American Journal of Nutrition* 35 (1935): 403–410.

Peace D., et al. "Self Selection of Food by Infants." *Journal of the Canadian Dietetic Association* 34 (1973): 191.

Story, M., and Brown, J. E. "Do Young Children Instinctively Know What to Eat? The Studies of Clara Davis Revisited." *New England Journal of Medicine* 316 (1987): 103–106.

The Development of Taste

Birch, L. L. "Effects of Peer Models' Food Choices and Eating Behaviors on Preschoolers' Food Preferences." *Child Development* 51 (1980): 489–496.

Birch, L. L., et al. "What Kind of Exposure Reduces Children's Food Neophobia?" *Appetite* 9 (1987): 171–178.

———. "Effects of Instrumental Consumption on Children's Food Preferences." *Appetite* 3 (1982): 125–134.

———. "I Don't Like It; I Never Tried It: Effects of Exposure on Two-year-old Children's Food Preference." *Appetite* 3 (1982): 353–360.

———. "The Influence of Social-affective Context on the Formation of Children's Food Preferences." *Child Development* 5 (1980): 856–861.

Floyd, B. L., et al. "Developing Good Food Habits in the Preschool Child. Humber College Day Care Centre - A Model." *Journal of the Canadian Dietetic Association* 40 (1979): 270–273.

Harper, L. V., et al. "The Effect of Adult's Eating on Young Children's Acceptance of Unfamiliar Foods." *Journal of Experimental Child Psychology* 20 (1975): 206–214.

Rozin, P., and Schiller, D. "The Nature and Acquisition of a Preference for Chili Pepper by Humans." *Motivation and Emotion* 4 (1980): 77–101.

Profiles of Preschoolers

Bates, Ames L., Ilg, F. L., and Chase, Haber C. *Your One-Year-Old*. New York: Delacorte, 1982.

———. *Your Two-Year-Old*. New York: Delacorte, 1976.

———. *Your Three-Year-Old, Your Four-Year-Old*. New York: Delacorte, 1976.

———. *Your Five-Year-Old*. New York: Dell, 1979.

Chery, A., and Sabry, J. "Portion Size of Common Foods Eaten by Children." *Journal of the Canadian Dietic Association* 45 (1984): 230–233.

Endres, J. B., and Rockwell, J. "Food Nutrition, and the Young Child." St. Louis: Mosby, 1980.

Network of the Federal/Provincial/Territorial Group on Nutrition and the National Institute of Nutrition. "Promoting Nutitional Health during the Preschool Years. Canadian Guidelines." Ottawa, 1989.

Different Diet, Different Challenge

Christoffel, K. "A Pediatric Perspective on Vegetarian Nutrition." *Clinical Pediatrics* 20 (1981): 632–643.

Dwyer, J., et al. "Growth in New Vegetarian Preschool Children Using the Jenss-Bayley Curve Fitting Technique." *American Journal of Clinical Nutrition* 37 (1983): 815–827.

Jacobs, C., and Dwyer, J. T. "Vegetarian Children; Appropriate and Inappropriate Diets." *American Journal of Clinical Nutrition* 48 (1988): 811–818.

Klaper, M. *Pregnancy, Children and the Vegan Diet.* Umatilla, Florida: Gentle World, 1987.

MacLean, W. C., and Graham, G. G. "Vegetarianism in Children." *American Journal of Disease in Childhood* 134 (1980): 513–519.

Rossouw, J. E. "Kwashiorkor in North America." *American Journal of Clinical Nutrition* 49 (1989): 588–592.

Sanders, T. A. B. "Growth and Development of British Vegan Children." *American Journal of Clinical Nutrition* 48 (1988): 822–825.

Truesdell, D. D., and Acosta P. "Feeding the Vegan Infant and Child." *Journal of the American Dietetic Association* 85 (1985): 837–840.

van Staveren, W. A., et al. "Food Consumption, Growth and Development of Dutch Children Fed on Alternative Diets." *American Journal of Clinical Nutrition* 48 (1988): 819–821.

Supplements

Barness, L. A. "Adverse Effects of Overdosage of Vitamins and Minerals." *Pediatrics in Review* 8 (1986): 20–24.

Committee on Nutrition, Academy of Pediatrics. "Vitamin and Mineral Supplement Needs in Normal Children in the United States." *Pediatrics* 66 (1980): 1015–1021.

———. "Fluoride Supplementation: Revised Dosage Schedule." *Pediatrics* 63 (1979): 150–152.

Dubick, M. A., and Rucker, R. B. "Dietary Supplements and Health Aids - A Critical Evaluation Part 1." *Journal of Nutrition Education* 15 (1983): 47–52.

Johnston, C. C., et al. "Calcium Supplementation and Increases in Bone Mineral Density in Children." *The New England Journal of Medicine* 327 (1992): 82–87.

Marshall, C. W. *Vitamins and Minerals.* Philadelphia: George F. Stickley, 1983.

Nutrition Committee, Canadian Paediatric Society. "Megavitamin and Megamineral Therapy in Childhood." *Canadian Medical Association Journal* 143 (1990): 1009–1013.

Allergies

Bahna, S. L., et al. "Food Allergy: Diagnosis and Treatment." *Annals of Allergy* 51 (1983): 574–580.

Bierman, W. C., et al. "Food Allergy." *Pediatrics in Review* 3 (1982): 213–220.

Bock, S. A. "Prospective Appraisal of Complaints of Adverse Reactions to Foods in Children during the First Three Years of Life." *Pediatrics* 79 (1987): 683–688.

Bock, S. A., et al. "Pattern of Food Hypersensitivity during Sixteen Years of Doubled-blind Placebo Controlled Food Challenge." *Journal of Pediatrics* 117 (1990): 561–567.

Crook, W. G. "Food Allergy, the Great Masquerader." *Pediatric Clinics of North America* 22 (1975): 227–239.

———. *Tracking Down Hidden Food Allergy.* Tennessee: Professional Books, 1978.

Denman, A. M., "Nature and Diagnosis of Food Allergy." *Proceedings of the Nutrition Societies* 38 (1979): 391–402.

Foucart, T. "Developmental Aspects of Food Sensitivity in Childhood." *Nutrition Reviews* 42 (1984): 98–104.

Leinhas, J. L., et al. "Food Allergy Challenges: Guidelines and Implications." *Journal of the American Dietetic Association* 87 (1987): 604–608.

Sampson, H. A., et al. "Fatal and Near-fatal Anaphylactic Reactions to Food in Children and Adolescents." *The New England Journal of Medicine* 327 (1992): 380–384.

Speer, F. "Multiple Food Allergy." *Annals of Allergy* 34 (1975): 71–76.

Anemia

Dallman, P. R., et al. "Iron Deficiency in Infancy and Childhood." *The American Journal of Clinical Nutrition* 37 (1980): 86–118.

———. "Prevalence and Causes of Anemia in the United States, 1976–1980." *American Journal of Clinical Nutrition* 39 (1984): 437–445.

Deinard, A., et al. "Iron Deficiency and Behavioral Defects." *Pediatrics* 68 (1981): 828–833.

Liebel, R. L. "Behavioral and Biochemical Correlates of Iron Deficiency." *Journal of the American Dietetic Association* 71 (1977): 398–404.

Lozoff, B. "Iron and Learning Potential in Childhood." *Bulletin of the New York Academy of Medicine* 10 (1989): 1050–1066.

Nutrition Committee, Canadian Paediatric Society. "Meeting the Iron Needs of Infants and Young Children; An Update." *Canadian Medical Association Journal* 11 (1991): 1451–1454.

Oski, F. A. "Unusual Manifestations of Iron Deficiency." *Nutrition & the MD* VIII (June 1982)

Oski, F. A., et al. "The Effects of Therapy on the Developmental Scores of Iron Deficient Infants." *Journal of Pediatrics* 92 (1978): 21–25.

Oski, F. A., and Stockman, J. A. "Anemia Due to Inadequate Iron Sources or Poor Iron Utilization." *Pediatrics Clinics of North America* 27 (1980): 237–252.

Pollitt, E., et al. "Significance of Bayley Scale Score Changes Following Iron Therapy." *Journal of Pediatrics* 92 (1978): 177–178.

Scrimshaw, N. "Iron Deficiency." *Scientific American* (October 1991): 46–52.

Atherosclerosis

Breslow, J. L. "Pediatric Aspects of Hyperlipidemia." *Pediatrics* 62 (1978): 510–520.

Canadian Consensus Conference on Cholesterol. Final Report. *Supplement to the Canadian Medical Association Journal* 139 (1988).

Glueck, C. J. "Cradle-to-Grave Atherosclerosis; High Density Lipoprotein Cholesterol." *Journal of the American College of Nutrition* 1 (1982): 41–48.

Morrisson, J. A., et al. "Parent-Child Association at Upper and Lower Ranges of Plasma Cholesterol and Triglyceride Levels." *Pediatrics* 62 (1978): 468–477.

National Cholesterol Education Program. "Report of the Expert Panel on Blood Cholesterol Levels in Children and Adolescents." *Pediatrics* 89 (1992): Supplement part 2.

Voller, R. D., and Strong, W. B. "Pediatric Aspects of Athersclerosis." *American Heart Journal* 101 (1981): 815–836.

Workshop Proceedings. "An Evaluation of the 1990 Nutrition Recommendations for Total Fat and Saturated Fat Intake for Children between the Ages of 2 and 18 Years." Toronto: Kush Medical Communications, 1991.

Constipation

Fitzgerald, J. F. "Constipation in Children." *Pediatrics in Review* 8 (1987): 299–302.

Freeman, N. V. "Faecal Soiling and Constipation in Children." *The Practitioner* 221 (1978): 333–337.

Gleghorn E. D., et al. "No-enema Therapy for Idiopathic Constipation and Encopresis." *Clinical Pediatrics* 30 (1990): 669–672.

Morcer, R. D. "Constipation." *Pediatric Clinics of North America* 14 (1967): 175–185.

Rappaport, L. A., et al. "The Prevention of Constipation and Encopresis: A Developmental Model and Approach." *Pediatric Clinics of North America* 33 (1986): 859–868.

Roach, J. J. "Constipation." *Journal of the National Medical Association* 70 (1978): 591–596.

Shaefer, C. E. "*Childhood Encopresis and Enuresis*." Chapter 2. *Bowel Physiology*. New York: Van Nortrand Reinhold Co.,1979.

Diarrhea

Charney, E. D., et al. "Intractable Diarrhea Associated with the Use of Sorbitol." *Journal of Pediatrics* 98 (1981): 157.

Cohen, S. A., et al. "Chronic Nonspecific Constipation: Dietary Relationship." *Pediatrics* 64 (1979): 402–407.

Hyams J. S., et al. "Carbohydrate Malabsorption following Fruit Juice Ingestion in Young Children." *Pediatrics* 82 (1988): 64–67.

Issenman, R. M., et al. "Are Chronic Digestive Complaints the Result of Abnormal Dietary Patterns?" *American Journal of Disease in Childhood* 141 (1987): 679–682.

Lifshitz, F., et al. "Role of Juice Carbohydrate Malabsorption in Chronic Nonspecific Diarrhea in Children." *The Journal of Pediatrics* 120 (1992): 825–829.

Lloyd-Still, J. D. "Chronic Diarrhea of Childhood and the Misuse of Elimination Diets." *Journal of Pediatrics* 95 (1979): 10–13.

Treem, W. R. "Chronic Nonspecific Diarrhea of Childhood." *Clinical Pediatrics* (July 1992): 413–419.

Walker-Smith, J. A. "Toddler's Diarrhea." *Archives of Disease in Childhood* 55 (1980): 329–330.

Gastroenteritis

Brown, K. H., et al. "Nutritional Management of Acute Diarrhea: An Appraisal of the Alternatives." *Pediatrics* 73 (1984):

Dupont, H. L., and Pickerings, L. K. *Infections of the Gastrointestinal Tract.* New York: Plenum Publishing Co., 1980.

Finberg, L., et al. "Oral Rehydration for Diarrhea." *Journal of Pediatrics* 101 (1982): 497–499.

Hamilton, J. R. "Dietary Fluids and Diarrhea in Babies." *Canadian Medical Association Journal* 121 (1979): 509–510.

Hirschorn, N. "The Treatment of Acute Diarrhea in Children. A Historical and Physiological Perspective." *American Journal of Clinical Nutrition* 33 (1980): 637–663.

Holdaway, M. D. "Management of Gastroenteritis in Early Childhood." *Drugs* 14 (1977): 383–389.

Hoyle, B., et al. "Breast-feeding and Food Intake Among Children with Acute Diarrheal Discare." *American Journal of Clinical Nutrition* 33 (1980): 2365–2371.

Hyams, J. S., et al. "Lactose Malabsorption Following Rotavirus Infection in Young Children." *Journal of Pediatrics* 99 (1981): 916–918.

Leung A. K. C., et al. "Acute Diarrhea in Children." *Postgraduate Medicine* 86 (1989): 161–170.

Snyder, J. "From Pedialyte to Popsicles: a Look at Oral Rehydration Therapy Used in the United States and Canada." *American Journal of Clinical Nutrition* 35 (1982): 157–161.

Sutton, R. E., et al. "Tolerance of Young Children with Severe Gastroenteritis to Dietary Lactose: A Controlled Study." *Canadian Medical Association Journal* 99 (1968): 980–982.

Wendland, B. E., and Arbus, G. S. "Oral Fluid Therapy: Sodium and Potassium Content and Osmolarity of Some Commercial 'Clear' Soups, Juices and Beverages." *Canadian Medical Association Journal* 121 (1979): 564–571.

Hyperactivity

Colquhoun, I., et al. "A Lack of Essential Fatty Acids as a Possible Cause of Hyperactivity in Children." *Medical Hypothesis* 7 (1981): 673–679.

Dickerson, J. W. T., et al. "Diet and Hyperactivity." *Journal of Human Nutrition* 34 (1980): 167–174.

Harper, P. H., et al. "Nutrient Intakes of Children on the Hyperkinesis Diet." *Journal of the American Dietetic Association* 73 (1978): 515–519.

Haslam R., et al. "Effects of Megavitamin Therapy on Children with Attention Deficit Disorders." *Pediatrics* 74 (1984): 103–110.

Kaplan, B. J., et al. "Dietary Replacement in Preschool-age Hyperactive Boys." *Pediatrics* 83 (1989): 7–17.

Lipton, M. A., et al. "Diet and Hyperkinesis — an Update." *Journal of the American Dietetic Association* 83 (1983): 132–134.

Mental Health Committee, Canadian Paediatric Society. "Hyperactivity in Children." *Canadian Medical Association Journal* 139 (1988): 211–212.

McNicol, J. "Diet and Behavior: Sense or Nonsense." Alberta Children's Hospital, 1983.

National Institutes of Health Consensus Development. "Conference Statement: Defined Diets and Childhood Hyperactivity." *American Journal of Clinical Nutrition* 37 (1983): 161–165.

Pipes, P. L. *Nutrition in Infancy and Childhood.* 4th ed. St. Louis: Mosby, 1989.

Rapp, D. *Allergies and the Hyperactive Child.* New York: Simon and Schuster, 1979.

Swanson, J. M., et al. "Food Dyes Impair Performance of Hyperactive Children on a Laboratory Learning Test." *Science* 207 (1980): 1485–1487.

Weiss, G., et al. "The Hyperactive Child Syndrome." *Science* 205 (1979): 1348–1354.

Weiss, B., et al. "Behavioral Responses to Artificial Food Colours." *Science* 207 (1980): 1487–1489.

Hypoglycemia

Liebman, B. "Hypoglycemia." *Nutrition Action* 7 (1980): 3–5.

Lafranchi, S. "Hypoglycemia of Infancy and Childhood." *Pediatric Clinics of North America* 34 (1987): 961–980.

"Special Report: Statement on Hypoglycemia." *Diabetes* 22 (1973): 137.

Lactose Intolerance

Barr, R. G., et al. "Recurrent Abdominal Pain of Childhood Due to Lactose Intolerance." *The New England Journal of Medicine* 300 (1979): 1449–1452.

Committee on Nutrition, American Academy of Pediatrics. "The Practical Significance of Lactose Intolerance in Children." *Pediatrics* 86 (1990): 643–644.

Kolars, J. C., et al. "Yogurt: An Autodigesting Source of Lactose." *The New England Journal of Medicine* 310 (1984): 1–3.

Lebenthal, E., et al. "Recurrent Abdominal Pain and Lactose Absorption in Children." *Pediatrics* 67 (1981): 828–832.

Lisker, R., et al. "Double Blind Study of Milk Lactose Intolerance in a Group of Rural and Urban Children." *American Journal of Clinical Nutrition* 33 (1980): 1049–1053.

Metz, G., et al. "Breath Hydrogen as Diagnostic Method for Hypolactasia." *Lancet* 1 (1975): 1155–1157.

Newcomer, A. D., and McGill, D. B. "Clinical Importance of Lactase Deficiency." *The New England Journal of Medicine* 310 (1984): 42–43.

Scrimshaw N. S., et al. "The Acceptability of Milk and Milk Products in Populations with a High Prevalence of Lactose Intolerance. *American Journal of Clinical Nutrition* 48 (suppl.) (1988): 1079–1159.

Obesity

Callaway, C. W., et al. "Relationship of Basal Metabolic Rates to Meal-Eating Patterns." 4th International Congress on Obesity: New York, 1983.

Committee on Nutrition, American Academy of Pediatrics. "Nutritional Aspects of Obesity in Infancy and Childhood." *Pediatrics* 68 (1981): 880–883.

Dietz, W. H. "Prevention of Childhood Obesity." *Pediatric Clinics of North America* 33 (1986): 823–833.

Dubois, S., et al. "An Examination of Factors Believed to Be Associated with Infantile Obesity." *American Journal of Clinical Nutrition* 32 (1979): 1997–2004.

Fritz, J. L., et al. "Preschoolers' Beliefs Regarding the Obese Individual." *Canadian Home Economics Journal* 32 (1982): 193–196.

Garrow, J. S. "Infant Feeding Obesity in Adults." *Bibliotheca Nutr. Dieta*, 26 (1978): 29–35.

Goldbloom, R. B. "Obesity in Childhood." *Kellogg Nutrition Symposium* (1976): 80–111.

Gorthmaker, S. L., et al. "Increasing Pediatric Obesity in the United States." *American Journal of Disease in Childhood* 141 (1987): 535–540.

Griffiths, M., and Payne, P. R. "Energy Expenditure in Small Children of Obese and Non-Obese Parents." *Nature* 260 (1976): 698–700.

Kolata, G. "Obese Children: A Growing Problem." *Science* 232 (April 1986): 20–21.

Leonard, C. P., et al. "Effects of a Weight-Control Program on Parent's Responses to Family Eating Situations." *Journal of the American Dietetic Association* 84 (1984): 424–428.

Myres, A. W. and Yeung, D. L. "Obesity in Infants: Significance Aetiology and Prevention." *Canadian Journal of Public Health* 70 (1979): 113–119.

Pomerance, H. H., et al. "The Relationship of Birth Size to the Rate of Growth in Infancy and Childhood." *American Journal of Clinical Nutrition* 39 (1984): 95–99.

Pugliese, M. T., et al. "Fear of Obesity." *New England Journal of Medicine* 309 (1983): 424–428.

———. "Fear of Obesity." *New England Journal of Medicine* 309 (1983): 513–518.

Saintonge, J., et al. "Are Macrosomic Babies a Risk for Future Obesity." *Journal of the Canadian Dietetic Association* 44 (1983): 132–138.

Sjostrom, L., and William-Olsson, T. "Prospective Studies on Adipose Tissue Development in Man." *International Journal of Obesity* 5 (1981): 597–604.

Unger, R., et al. "Childhood Obesity: Medical and Familial Correlates and Age of Onset." *Clinical Pediatrics* 29 (1990): 368–373.

Vobecky, J. S., et al. "Nutrient Intake Patterns and Nutritional Status with Regard to Relative Weight in Early Infancy." *American Journal of Clinical Nutrition* 38 (1983): 730–738.

Weil, W. B. "Obesity in Children." *Pediatrics in Review* 3 (1981): 180–189.

Wolman, P. W. "Feeding Practices in Infancy and Prevalence of Obesity in Preschool Children." *Journal of the American Dietetic Association* 84 (1984): 436–438.

Tooth Decay

Beagley, G. M. "Nursing-Bottle Syndrome." *Canadian Dietetic Association Journal* 39 (1978): 25–27.

Bibby, G. G. "The Cariogenicity of Snack Food and Confections." *Journal of the American Dental Association* 90 (1975): 121–132.

Caliendo, M. A. *Nutrition and Preventive Health Care.* New York: Macmillan, 1981.

Chudakov, B. K. "Sugar in Medications: the Covert Contributor to Dental Disease." *Canadian Pharmaceutical Journal* 117 (1984): 12–14.

Cudzinorvski, L. "Le Syndrome du biberon." *L'Union médicale du Canada* 109 (1980): 853–855.

Feizal, R. J., et al. "Dental Caries Potential of Liquid Medications." *Pediatrics* 68 (1981): 416–419.

Koranyi, K., et al. "Nursing Bottle Weaning and Prevention of Dental Caries: A Survey of Pediatricians." *Pediatric Dentistry* 13 (1991): 32–34.

McCormack-Brown, K. R., and McDermott, R. J. "Dental Caries: Selected Factors of Children at Risk." *The Dental Assistant* 60 (1991): 10–14.

Navia, V. M. "Prospects for Prevention of Dental Caries: Dietary Factors." *Journal of the American Dental Association* 87 (1973)1010–1012.

Nizel, A. E. "Preventing Dental Caries: The Nutritional Factors." *Pediatric Clinics of North America* 24 (1977): 141–155.

Pinkerton, R. E., et al. "Preventing Dental Caries." *American Family Physician* 23 (1981): 167–170.

Sclavos S., et al. "Future Caries Development in Children with Nursing Bottle Caries." *Journal of Pedodontics* 13 (1988): 1–10.

Microwaves, Barbecues, and Pressure Cookers

Hoffmann, C. J., et al. "Effects of Microwave Cooking and Reheating on Nutrients and Food Systems: A Review of Recent Studies." *Journal of the American Dietetic Association* 85 (1985): 922–926.

Klein, B. "Retention of Nutrients in Microwave-cooked Foods." *Contemporary Nutrition* 14 (1989):

Rechcigl, M. *Handbook of Nutritive Value of Processed Food.*: Boca Raton, Florida:CRC Press, 1982.

Fast Foods

Palik, B. "Qu'en est-il du fast food? Protégez-vous." (mai 1984): 21–26.

Zlotkin, S. H., "Controverse au sujet de la nutrition en 1984." *Medécine Moderne du Canada* 39 (1984): 443–448

Canned Foods

Mahaffey, K. R. "Nutritional Factors in Lead Poisoning." *Nutrition Reviews* 39 (1984): 353–362.

Schaffner, R. M. "Lead in Canned Foods." *Food Technology* (December 1981): 60–64.

Food Colorings

Health and Welfare Canada, Health Protection Branch. "Colouring Agents in Drugs." Information Letter 634 (1982)

Silbergeld, E. K., and Anderson, S. M. "Artificial Food Colors and Childhood Behavior Disorders." *Bulletin of the New York Academy of Medicine* 58 (1982): 275–295.

Swanson, J. M., et al. "Food Dyes Impair Performance of Hyperactive Children on a Laboratory Learning Test." *Science* 207 (1980): 1485–1487.

Weiss, B., et al. "Behavior Responses to Artificial Food Colors." *Science* 207 (1980): 1487–1489.

Salt

Khaw, K. T., et al. "Dietary Potassium and Blood Pressure in a Population." *American Journal of Clinical Nutrition* 39 (1984): 963–968.

Mattes, R. D. "Salt Taste and Hypertension: A Critical Review of the Literature." *Journal of Chronic Diseases* 37 (1984): 195–208.

McCarron, D. A., et al. "Assessment of Nutritional Correlates of Blood Pressure." *Annals of Internal Medicine* 98 (1983): 715–719.

———. "Blood Pressure and Nutrient Intake in the United States." *Science* 224 (1984): 1392–1398.

Wallis, C. "Salt: A New Villain?" *Time* (March 15, 1982):66–77

Whitten, C. F., and Stewart, R. A. "The Effect of Dietary Sodium in Infancy on Blood Pressure and Related Factors." *Acta Pædiatrica Scandinavica*, suppl. 279 (1980): 1–17.

Sweeteners

"Aspartame and Other Sweeteners." *The Medical Letter*, 24 (Janvier 1982).

Yokogoshi, H., et al. "Effects of Aspartame and Glucose Administration on Brain and Plasma Levels of Large Neutral Amino and Brain 5-Hydroxyindoles." *American Journal of Clinical Nutrition* 40 (1984): 1–7.

List of Tables

Index of Recipes

Recipes without Meat

Cheese Fondue,   *149*
Fettuccine Florentine,   *148*
Grilled Cheese Sandwich,   *150*
Lentil and Apple Soup,   *158*
Minute Pizza,   *157*
Spinach Quiche,   *161*
Vegetable Pie,   *164*
Wild Zucchini,   *146*

Recipes without Sugar

Apple and Almond Custard,   *169*
Miracle Compote,   *166*
Peanut Butter Squares,   *126*
Prune Juice Jelly,   *172*
Spring Compote,   *167*
Sunny Date and Apricot Jelly   *173*

Recipes without Wheat

Banana and Almond Muffins,   *174*
Buckwheat Pancakes,   *127*
Granola Special,   *128*
Peanut Butter Squares,   *126*
Shrimp Paella,   *151*

Recipes without Milk or Dairy Products

Almond and Sesame Milk,   *180*
Almond Milk (concentrated),   *181*
Banana and Almond Muffins,   *174*
Bran Muffins,   *176*
Buckwheat Pancakes,   *127*

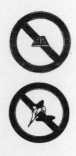

Recipes without Chocolate

Recipes without Corn

Recipes without Eggs

Recipes with a Lot of Vegetables

Recipes for Breakfast

Fish Recipes

Recipes for the Barbecue

Index

Cinnamon, allergy to, 40
Citrus fruits, allergy to, 40
Citrus red no. 2, 105
Colic, lactose intolerance, 75
Constipation, 55–59, 113
  acute, 55
  allergies, 40
  chronic, 56
  definition of, 55
  description of, 55
  diet high and low in dietary
    fiber, 58, 59
  effects on health, 55
  incidence of, 55
  laxatives and enemas, 57
  prevention of, 57
  treatment (increase of dietary
    fiber in the diet), 57, 59
Corn, allergy to, 40
Corn syrup, high in fructose, 113
Cramps, 69
  allergies, 40
  lactose intolerance, 60

Desserts, preferences, 3
Diabetes, 80
Diarrhea, allergies, 40
  lactose intolerance, 75
Diets,
  elimination, for allergies,
    41–54
  high and low in fiber, 58–59
  high and low in lactose, 78
  high and moderate in fat,
    53–54
  high in and without sugar, 74,
    91
  lacto-ovo-vegetarian, 32
  low and high in calories, 86
  low and high in iron, 49
  omnivorous, 31
  prevention for obesity, 84–85

recovery to eliminate chronic
    diarrhea, 62
  recovery for gastroenteritis, 66
  vegan, 33

Eating habits of the very young,
    3–4
Eczema, allergies, 40
Eggs, allergy to, 40
Elimination diet, 41–45
Erythrosine (food color), 105
Essential fatty acids, 68, 108

Fast foods, 100–102
  hidden fat in foods, 101
  hidden salt in foods, 102
Fast green (food color), 105
Fasting, 64
Fats, 108–111
  foods containing hidden fat,
    110–111
  foods high in saturated, 52
  hidden in fast food, 101
Feingold, Dr. Ben, 68, 105
Fiber, 113, 202
  Diets high and low in, 58–59
  increase intake of, 57
  in vegetables, 27
Fish, 21, 108
Floss, 89
Fluoride, 196
  recommended quantities, 89
  supplements of, 35, 89, 196
  use of, 89
Folacin, 191
Foods, acceptance of, 10–12
  canned, 103–104
  cholesterol in certain, 52
  containing hidden fat, 110–11
  containing hidden sugar,
    115–17
  containing one or more food

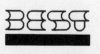

PRINTED IN CANADA